The Healing Church

The Healing Church

Practical Programs for Health Ministries

Abigail Rian Evans

United Church Press
Cleveland, Ohio

Library of Congress Cataloging-in-Publication Data

Evans, Abigail Rian.
  The healing church : practical programs for health ministries / Abigail Rian Evans.
    p. cm.
  Companion to: Redeeming marketplace medicine.
  Includes bibliographical references and index.
  ISBN 0-8298-1340-3 (pbk. : alk. paper)
  1. Medicine—Religious aspects—Christianity.   2. Medical care—Moral and ethical aspects.   3. Pastoral medicine.   I. Title.
BT732.2.E833   1999
261.5'61—dc21   99-34476
                                                                   CIP

To my grandchildren and daughters-in-law,
who have brought hope, healthiness, and happiness
to me and to so many others:

Kathy Barton	*Mary Tiebout*	*Wendy Hoadley*
Alex, Sara,	*Johanna*	*Elizabeth*
and Thomas	*and Eli*	

Cheryl Coyner
"Mother" for many years to
the American Boychoir youngsters

Contents

Preface

Good health has been a primary goal in every society throughout history. All people crave healing, whether of physical, emotional, or spiritual sickness. Almost $1 trillion is spent each year on drugs, doctors, quacks, and healers. Cures have been sought in almost every conceivable form, from bloodletting and incantations, to healing services and prayer meetings, to sophisticated drugs and refined surgical procedures.

As a missionary in Brazil in the 1960s, I witnessed firsthand how people suffered from poor health because of malnutrition, poverty, and the lack of necessary medical resources. Watching people eat from garbage cans, drink unclean water, and die of complications from untreated parasites seared on my conscience the need for the church to engage in a health ministry to body, mind, and spirit. Upon returning to the United States to work in Appalachia, New York City, Washington, D.C., and southern Virginia, and more recently as I have traveled through the United Kingdom, I have seen economic exploitation, workaholism, stress, and incurable illness among the people of God. My conscience and my call to ministry exhort me to write this book about the church's opportunities and responsibilities for health ministries.

We live in an environment of failed health care reform, marketplace medicine, and rising health care costs. Unfortunately, the contemporary understanding of healing and healers emphasizes disease and illness rather than health promotion and illness prevention. The medical model dominates our interpretation of healers as those who respond to a crisis rather than prevent it. An important link is missing between the medical establishment and the other health institutions in our community. Allopathic medicine and hospital-based care alone cannot adequately address these problems.

The best corrective to this dominant medical model and managed health care may be the reemergence of the church as a major health care provider. The church may take its place alongside the hospital as a center for the promotion of health and the treatment of illness. In prophetic contrast to the medical model, it can highlight the educational and preventive responsibilities of the healer.

As I argued in my companion book, *Redeeming Marketplace Medicine: A Theology of Health Care*, the church can function as a health institution and a healing community by basing its ministry on a broader definition of health as wholeness, sickness as brokenness, and healers as those persons who assist us toward health. The church is the corporate expression of the individual Christian's calling to a healing ministry. It can contribute to our personal movement toward health as well as furnish part of a concrete health care system.

It is not so much the institutional structure, but the communal nature of the church that makes it a force for healing. The ministry of healing is not optional, but a binding commitment to confront evil in the form of sickness; it forms an integral part of the whole life of the church.

This book, by showing how the Christian faith and the church can offer concrete solutions, encourages pastors, church members, health care professionals, and church and hospital personnel to join in partnership to revolutionize the health care system and reposition the church in its historic healing ministry. It is written for those in the American and British context; my hope is that it will be especially helpful to health care professionals to link their Christian faith to a health and healing ministry. In addition, its descriptions of successful health ministries programs are meant to inspire and equip church groups to become concretely involved in this reenvisioning and revolution of our health care delivery systems. This book centers on God's calling that health should be the agenda of the church; that there are a variety of resources available for health ministry; and that healing is needed in all seasons of life, not just in the crises of physical illness.

The four main theses of this book are as follows: (1) the church's involvement in health care is based on its historic healing ministry, which forms an important base for assessing current healing ministries; (2) the fullness of time for the church to recover its healing ministry is now, because of the changing nature of illness, the crisis in health care, the expansion of health care practices, the rediscovery of the link between spirituality and health, and scientific studies of the effects of religious beliefs and practices on good health; (3) the church's health ministry can be classified in four general categories—liturgical/sacramental/devotional, educational, support and advocacy, and direct health care; and (4) the contemporary healing ministry of the church is emerging as "health ministry," perhaps considered a new discipline.

A few words about health ministry as a discipline might be in order because the term also refers to programs, that is, "health ministries." The medicine/religion dialogue, sacramental and charismatic healing ministries, bioethics, medical missions work, the establishment of the Wholistic Health Centers, Inc., and the Carter and Park Ridge Centers, the rise of complementary health care practices, and most recently, the public interest in spirituality and health all contribute to what could be regarded as a new discipline—health ministry. Working within these different streams from the 1970s to the 1990s has convinced me that collectively they help to frame and define this new discipline.

First, my medical ethics studies with Paul Ramsey in the 1970s, whose conceptualization of this field as a Methodist layman, influenced by Catholic moral theology, helped me to understand the importance of a theological perspective in the developing discipline of bioethics. Later my work with William F. May, a theological ethicist, Presbyterian minister, and now the Cary M. Maguire Professor of Ethics at Southern Methodist University, inspired and invigorated me to look at the church's contribution to bioethics and health ministries.

Subsequent to founding and directing National Capital Presbytery Health Ministries in the 1980s and serving as director of new programs and senior staff associate at the Kennedy Institute of Ethics at Georgetown University in Washington, D.C., I moved between the worlds of medicine, church, government, social service agencies, and academia. I saw how they all contributed to this new discipline of health ministry. My involvements included serving as an ethicist on the Institutional Review Board at the Neurology Institute at the National Institutes of Health; becoming a member of the U.S. Government Office for Substance Abuse Prevention Religious Task Force, and of the international network on addiction prevention of the Christian Medical Commission of the World Council of Churches; being involved in the Washington, D.C., Kidney Foundation organ donor project; serving as a member of the Clinton Health Care Reform Task Force; and working with numerous other agencies that were discovering how fruitful a partnership with the church could be. While being involved in these various endeavors, I was serving as an interim pastor at different Presbyterian churches and preaching at dozens of different congregations. I mention this because it was precisely as a pastor that I saw the importance of a collaborative approach between the church and other agencies and disciplines to meet members' health-related needs.

Through these experiences and those of others, I began to understand that health ministry was a new form of the church's healing ministry. However, because it synthesizes so many other disciplines, it appears to be a new discipline as well as a style of programming. Although considerable research and writing have been devoted to these separate subjects, my desired contribution is to help frame this newly emerging discipline, which works at the interface of theology, ethics, medicine, culture, and ecclesiology.

Within this discipline, health ministries programs can be defined as broad-based approaches to health care that are sponsored, located, or initiated by a community of faith or most generally a church. By describing four categories of health ministry "programs," I offer a vision of the church's ministry as more than healing services, but inclusive of a variety of health-related programs.

May this book, along with its companion volume, *Redeeming Marketplace Medicine: A Theology of Health Care*, become a resource at this very crucial time of reframing the health care system as well as reenergizing the church for effective and important programs in the life of the community, the nation, and the world.

Acknowledgments

A book may have a single author listed, but many important people make its creation possible. I have been blessed with numerous wonderful friends, family members, assistants, and colleagues who have helped in countless ways. First, I would like to thank my family—my sisters Marian Hays and Roanne Pulliam, for their special help, and my sons Stephen, Nato, Matthew, and Thomas, who have encouraged me in the long process of writing my book. Second, my administrative and research assistants Janice Miller, James Lynch, Lisa Wells, and Jane Brady, who have helped in countless ways in the book production, finding important references and statistics, as well as Jane Ferguson who, in addition to these tasks, assisted very effectively in interviewing health ministries staff and clarifying conceptual issues. I am also grateful to Tim Staveteig and Kim Sadler of The Pilgrim Press and United Church Press, whose confidence and encouragement have facilitated the writing and completion of this and my companion book.

Appreciation also goes to Princeton Theological Seminary, which graciously gave me the sabbatical necessary for my research, and the Lilly Foundation, which provided the faculty research grant to visit effective health ministries programs around the country. Thanks go as well to the staff of those programs who introduced me to their exciting and crucial work of ministering to people's health-related needs in many innovative ways. The Presbyterian Church (USA), Office of Health Ministries, under Dave Zuverink and James Tibbett, provided a grant to Princeton Theological Seminary to pilot health ministries at the seminary. For the last dozen years, this office has taken a leadership role in health ministries. In addition, National Capital Presbytery, under the leadership of Ed White, sponsored and supported, along with the Vidda Foundation, one of the first health ministries presbytery programs in the country in the 1980s, enabling me to learn through doing health ministries.

I am especially indebted to Norma Small and Ann Solari Twadell for their helpful insights about the parish nurse program. My hope is that this book may especially be a resource for parish nurses and other health ministers as well as pastors and church members who are searching for new ways to carry forth Christ's healing ministry. Finally, I am grateful to all those persons named and unnamed who have enhanced my health in its broadest meaning even in the midst of my serious illnesses, giving me a glimpse of God's grace and healing through their deeds and words of love and kindness.

The Church's Historic Role in Health and Healing

The healing ministry of the Christian church has been sadly misunderstood and often relegated to the fringes of the church and to various sectarian groups. It is not some occasional activity or special project—nor is it random, breathtaking events that happen at Lourdes or miracle cures that touch only small numbers of people. The ministry of the church as a health institution is at the heart of its whole mission and should permeate every part of its mission. The communal nature of the church makes it a force for healing.

Given the church's historical commitment to health and healing, many people wonder if today's church is being true to its call to heal. Although the church offers the sacraments, holds worship services, and preaches the Word, the fourth mark of the church—healing the sick—has not been practiced in the full sense of a healing ministry. In many cases, because of fear of abuse, we have neglected Christ's charge to his disciples to heal. Often healing has been totally spiritualized so that its physical dimension has been lost; but healing and saving have the same root, and the concepts should be understood wholistically—healing of mind, body, and spirit.[1] The history of these concepts becomes an important base for assessing current healing practices and appreciating the struggles Christians have always faced in implementing Christ's call to heal.

The history of the church's healing ministry is uneven at best, changing with the theological emphases of different periods. The following overview does not do justice to the subtle nuances of the Christian healing ministry but provides a context for understanding contemporary health ministry. Fortunately, under Martin Marty's visionary leadership, Project

Ten, begun at the Chicago-based Park Ridge Center, has produced four-teen volumes on the medicine/religion interface in all the major religious traditions as well as two summary volumes.[2]

The purpose here is not to give a comprehensive review of the whole of the church's involvement but to touch on a few key themes which show that church-based health care forms a direct historical line from Jesus' healing ministry; it is not just a twentieth-century phenomenon.[3] There are four principal strains of this history: sacramental healing in the Roman Catholic and Anglican Churches; the development of hospitals beginning in the monasteries; the medical mission work of later centuries; and the rise of contemporary health ministries.

The church's healing ministry can be divided into different periods that illustrate these emphases: (1) Jesus' healing ministry, the apostolic and patristic periods; (2) the founding of hospitals during the Middle Ages; (3) the medicine/religion split, starting with the Renaissance/Reformation; (4) the medical mission movement in the nineteenth century to mid-twentieth century; (5) the religion/medicine and bioethical quandary debates in the 1950s–70s; and more recently, (6) the development of health ministries.

NEW TESTAMENT PERIOD—JESUS' HEALING SHOWS CONCERN FOR TOTAL HEALTH

During Jesus' ministry, God was viewed as the source of health but also as One who could use sickness and suffering for spiritual growth. Jesus cured people of all kinds of diseases, even death itself, sometimes by touching the person and simply by speaking a word. Historian and patristic scholar Evelyn Frost suggests that Christ's power over natural forces was displayed (1) in direct relation to persecution, empowering followers to withstand and even be joyful during the tortures of the persecutions; (2) in connection with demons, providing a cure before science had named diseases that the Bible attributed to satanic forces, and transforming the lives of those relieved of their torment; and (3) in relation to physical disease and death whereby the church considered it "a great sin not to heal sufferers" and frequently mentioned the use of gifts of healing. As evidence of Christ's power to heal physical disease, Frost points out that the healings were "well known to non-Christians . . . , often leading to their conversion" and that the Roman authorities were "able to attest to these healings."[4]

That Jesus considered healing to be central to his ministry is borne out by his ordering of healing as one of the top three duties, next to preaching and teaching, that he delegated to his twelve disciples. Jesus sent out the disciples two by two with "authority over the unclean spirits" (Mark 6:7).

Matthew 10:1 elaborates that the disciples were equipped not only to cast out unclean spirits but also to "cure every disease and every sickness." Luke 9:1–2 mentions Jesus' mandate to the disciples "to cure diseases," "to proclaim the realm of God and to heal." Part of this healing included visitation of the sick, based on Matthew 25:36: "I was sick and you took care of me."[5]

APOSTOLIC AGE—MIRACULOUS HEALINGS AND RITES

Miraculous healings were common during the apostolic period. They witnessed to the continuity and the importance of Christ's healing ministry and to the authenticity of the gospel that the apostles preached. Members of the early church were convinced of Christ's victory over powers and principalities (Eph. 6:12) and similarly regarded themselves as wrestling against them.[6] The gift of healing, given by Christ to the church, was used to testify to the resurrection and the current realization of God's reign. Morris Maddocks notes that the healing ministry of the early church "evoked faith in Jesus' mighty work of death/resurrection and so led to belief in him as Saviour and Lord."[7]

Many extraordinary healings are featured in the Acts of the Apostles, which records nineteen healings: three by Peter (3:2; 5:15; 9:32, 37), one by John and Peter (3:2), nine by Paul (14:3, 8, 19; 15:12; 19:11; 20:9; 28:3, 8, 9), one by Philip (8:7), one by Ananias (9:17), and four by the apostles in general (2:43; 5:12, 16; 8:13). There is no record of Jesus anointing or of the disciples anointing after Pentecost. However, anointing the sick with oil had already been practiced by the disciples before the Ascension (Mark 6:13).

Healing the sick and preaching the Word were inevitably linked to the in-breaking of the reign of God. Maddocks notes, "Confrontation with illness was not for [the apostles] . . . a stumbling block to the new life in Christ which they were proclaiming. Rather they accepted it as *ho kairos*, the opportunity given by God to proclaim [God's] wonderful works and give [God] glory. It was a confirmation of the word they were entrusted to preach."[8] Of the healing style of the apostles, Maddocks adds that "they did not make a fuss about it; they merely got on with it."[9]

James 5 as the Origin of the Rite of Healing

The classic description of the rite of healing in the early church is found in James's epistle. The James 5 passage has traditionally been understood as the aegis of the rite of healing. This particular scripture appears at the end of a passage that is principally addressing moral and ethical practices rather than precise theological formulations:

> Are any among you suffering? They should pray. Are any cheerful? They should sing songs of praise. Are any among you sick? They should call for the elders of the church and have them pray over them, anointing them with oil in the name of God. The prayer of faith will save the sick, and God will raise them up; and anyone who has committed sins will be forgiven. Therefore confess your sins to one another, and pray for one another, so that you may be healed. The prayer of the righteous is powerful and effective. (James 5:13–16)

A key term in this James passage is the reference to "elders" (*presbyteros*). Palestinian Jews used the word "elders" (*zeqenim*) for those who handled sacred functions (m. Aboth 1:1),[10] but the elders referenced here are linked with the Christian church with one of their specific functions being praying for the sick.[11] An important dimension is the presence of the elders—not just the priest but a group of elders—as a sign of the love of the community.[12] It seems no accident that the James passage refers to elders in the plural when giving the instruction for the administration of the anointing. Sickness and dying, then, are reintroduced within the community of believers. Hence, instead of the sick person being isolated, as modern medicine has done by removing the person from her community at a time when isolation is one of the biggest fears, she is put back into the center of the community.

At the time James was written, oil was commonly used for healing the sick in both the pagan and the Judeo-Christian worlds. In everyday life, oil was applied as a soothing lotion for athletes as well as perfume or ointment for the body. It was also used in the anointing of kings. Here its purpose was both to save (*sozein*) and to restore (*egeirein*). Most scholars argue that these terms indicate both bodily and spiritual healing. Since *egeirein* can also mean "to rise up on the last day" or "to rise up from the sickbed" or both, the meaning cannot be determined from the context alone. The "saving and raising up" in James 5 refers to the integration of sickness within one's Christian life and bringing to bear the meaning of Christ's death and resurrection in the life of the patient. The anointing is a sign of the strengthening and comfort of Christ. The death of Christ, however, has meaning only in relation to the resurrection. Catholic scholars see a further link between the anointing of the sick with oil and the forgiveness of sins.[13] This anointing can bring an infusion of power and healing force for a short time or simply sustain the person.[14]

The James passage emphasizes the saving of the sick with the prayer of faith, accompanied by anointing. Did James consider this anointing to be remedial or religious? According to Charles Gusmer, the James passage indicates that the elders, not those with special gifts of healing, exercise the general commission to heal.[15] Was it a sacrament conveying sanctifying grace *ex opere operato* or a sacramental provision of supernatural means for the recovery of health?

PATRISTIC PERIOD—GIFTS OF HEALING AND WHOLISTIC HEALTH

Moving from the Christian Scriptures' accounts of healing to the patristic, a wholistic perspective of healing continued. Healing was widely practiced in the church during the patristic period, from praying in God's name and signing of the cross to "exorcism, laying on of hands and anointing with oil."[16] Frost holds that the ante-Nicene church was transformed by the power of the risen Christ, whose victory extended to the preservation of the whole human person—soul, mind, and body.

Salvation and Health—Twin Concepts

Many of the ante-Nicene writers continued the scriptural emphasis of the connection between health and salvation. As was extensively discussed in my companion book, *Redeeming Marketplace Medicine*, health and salvation were not identical but twin concepts signifying wholeness. Ignatius (ca. 35–ca. 107 C.E.), for example, provides evidence outside the Christian Scriptures that the early church viewed salvation wholistically. He implores his second-century audience "thoroughly pure and self-controlled, [to] remain body and soul united to Jesus Christ,"[17] and further advises them to "stand firmly by the orders of the Lord and the apostles, so that 'whatever you do, you may succeed' in body and soul."[18]

Irenaeus (ca. 130–ca. 200 C.E.), Origen (ca. 185–ca. 254 C.E.), and Tertullian (160–220 C.E.) were familiar with the *Shepherd of Hermas*, a respected, widely read second-century record of five visions from God, reportedly to a Christian and slave in Rome.[19] The *Shepherd* cites the great joy of relieving people of their suffering. It reflects the Hebrew understanding of the integration of body and spirit rather than the Gnostic dualism familiar at the time: "Also take heed that it be not instilled into thy mind that this body perishes, and thou abuse it to any lust. For if thou shalt defile thy body, thou shalt also at the same time defile the Holy Spirit; and if thou shalt defile the Holy Spirit, thou shalt not live."[20]

Patristic writers such as Cyprian (d. 258) had a similarly wholistic under-standing of health and believed that those who refused to do penance or confess their sins would be possessed by unclean spirits.[21] Although John Crowlesmith asserts that Cyprian had a wholistic understanding of health, he nevertheless undervalues Cyprian's principal concern with dis-obedience to God leading to punishment in the form of sickness.[22] Further evidence of the ante-Nicene Father's wholistic view of health comes from the understanding that Holy Communion "[nourished] the body as well as the soul."[23] The ante-Nicene church even called the sacraments "the medicine of life," which Crowlesmith insists "must be taken as applying to the whole [person]."[24]

Gifts and Forms of Healing

The early church regarded the ministry of healing as central to the life and work of the church because the goodness of the body was affirmed. The human being was a unity of body, mind, and spirit. Healing became sacra-mental and was combined with anointing and exorcism.

Justin Martyr (ca. 100–ca. 165 C.E.) speaks of the gift of healing as one of the charismata still received in the church and refers to the early Christians' responsibility to care for the sick at their own expense.[25] Irenaeus of Lyons refers to such works of healing as "giving sight to the blind and hearing to the deaf; casting out demons; curing the lame, the paralytic and all physical ills; and raising the dead."[26]

During the patristic period there was a strong belief in miracles, although the more traditional Protestant view would refute this by con-tending that miraculous healing ceased with the apostolic age. Charles Harris remarks that in early times the Christian churches were referred to as "temples of healing."[27] For the most part, however, exorcisms were much more dominant in the patristic writings than miraculous healings, which still had a place. Demons were believed to inhabit places as well as people.[28] The prayers for the sick were heavily weighted toward the casting out of demons.[29]

Deacons were designated to serve the sick and to inform the bishop to pray over them. Healings took place by prayer, invocation of God's name, signing of the cross, exorcism, laying on of hands, anointing with oil, and a visit from the bishop to a sick person's house.[30] In fact, the *Canons of Hippolytus* mentions the charism of healing as a qualification for being a candidate for ordination.[31] The ordination prayers asked for the gifts of healing and exorcism to be bestowed upon the person. Of course, the gift of healing could be received by anyone, but if someone received this gift, it was a sign of a purity of life, hence one of the confirming signs of being called to the priesthood. In addition, all catechumens were expected to participate in the visitation of the sick, and a steward was to be established for the express purpose of caring for the sick.[32]

Theophilus of Antioch (later second century) cited divine healing from sickness as a proof of the power of the resurrection.[33] Tertullian referenced a number of exorcisms and even an anointing of the pagan emperor Severus with oil.[34] Though it is too early in the history of the church to consider this unction, most scholars agree that the earliest liturgical source for the consecration of oil for the sick is from the early third century. The oil was thought to have power to strengthen the body, the soul, and the mind.[35]

POST-CONSTANTINIAN PERIOD— SACRAMENT AND SUPERSTITION

In the post-Constantinian period three principal dimensions influenced the healing ministry of the church: political, cultural, and theological. The political realities were that as a state religion much of Christianity's healing power was weakened. The church's role was institutionalized.

The Roman culture blurred with Christianity, causing the use of charms, amulets, relics, and pilgrimages to holy places to predominate the healing ministry. St. Augustine writes extensively about the miraculous cures of blindness, fistulas, cancer, gout, malignant spirits, and paralysis by holy men of God after physicians had failed to work any cures. However, the "miracles" were connected with shrines and so forth. He recounts the story of a small boy who had been crushed by a cart. The boy's mother placed him in a shrine to St. Stephen, and he was completely cured with no sign of injury. Another story explains how the garment of a dying child was placed in the shrine, prayers were said, and the child was healed.[36]

The emerging theology of this time was that God sent sickness and used it for God's own purposes. In addition, the Protestant church taught that there was a certain period for miracles, which God later withdrew. "Christian healing then remained a 'spiritual' matter until the revival of interest in Christian bodily healing in the present century."[37] However, Stephen Pattison, a British pastoral theologian, criticizes this dispensationalist view since all through history Christians have seen a role for faith in healing. For example, pilgrimages, visits to saints' tombs or holy wells, and other vehicles for Christian healing were pursued, indicating more than "one mode" of Christian healing.[38] Frost takes a somewhat different view, arguing that the erosion of the church's powerful ministry of healing is shown by the veneration of the relics of the saints and pilgrimages to sacred shrines.

During the Dark Ages from 500 to 800 C.E., although the practices were full of superstition and magic, a belief in Christ's power remained. There are many fascinating stories about the use of relics and amulets of saints' bones and fabled pieces of the cross as well as pilgrimages to the Holy Land, which underscored the profound desire to be in the presence of Christ. This shift from God to holy relics was also due to the church's emphasis on the soul rather than the body. Since the church no longer had a principal interest in the body, the common folk turned to magic and superstition for physical healing.

Development of the Sacrament of Healing

During the post-Constantinian period, however, the rite of healing took on a sacramental and spiritualized meaning. It was referenced in the third to the fifth centuries' liturgical texts and from the fifth to the eighth centuries in patristic texts. Of prime importance was the consecration of the "matter" of the sacrament, in this instance the "oil."[39] The liturgy included a prayer of *epiclesis*, which called upon God to send the Holy Spirit to change the substance of the element. At that time it was not necessary for a priest to administer the sacraments or for a bishop to consecrate the oil. With the *Letter of Innocent I* (416 C.E.), the foundation for the administration of this sacrament was established. This letter is a reply to the bishop of Decentius of Gubbio who had asked Innocent's advice concerning the anointing of the sick by a bishop. The norms governing the administration of the sacrament were the consecration of the oil by the local bishop; the administration of the sacrament by Christians to one another, but preferably by the bishops; and the exclusion from the sacrament of anyone who needed "penance." (At that time there were not seven sacraments.)[40]

Although this period presented many changes to the church's views on health and healing, the sacrament of healing continued as an important part of the church's ministry of healing. Cesarius of Arles (503–43 C.E.), bishop of Provence, preached numerous sermons about the sacrament of anointing. He indicated that it was for use not only with serious illnesses but also with all kinds of sickness. Priests as well as bishops could consecrate the sacramental oil. Its efficacy was a result of prayer and a deep confidence in its results. Up to the end of the eighth century there was still no fixed rite of anointing, but there was consecration of the sacramental oil.[41]

MIDDLE AGES—THE FOUNDING OF HOSPITALS
AND THE SACRAMENT OF EXTREME UNCTION

During the Middle Ages there were two principal aspects to the healing ministry—the establishment of hospitals and the development of the sacrament of extreme unction. Although most scholars attribute the rise of hospitals to the monastic movement, James McGilvray believes the actual impetus for Christians to become involved in establishing hospitals should be traced to Emperor Constantine's withdrawal in 335 c.e. of "official recognition of Asclepius which had served both as temples and as refuges for the sick."[42] By some accounts, Constantine's mother, Helena, stepped up to fill in the gap by helping other Christians found hospitals,[43] following in the tradition of the first-century Christians who had opened their homes to the sick. The hospital of St. Basil in Caesarea founded in 369 c.e. is an illustration of this desire to help as is the Christian hospital at Constantinople, where two deaconesses nursed the sick.[44] Fabiola, a wealthy Roman matron, endowed a church-related hospital in Rome in 390 c.e. During this same period, St. Ephraim (ca. 306–73 c.e.) fled from his contemplative solitude to heed the cry of the distressed at "plague-stricken" Edessa, where he founded a three-hundred-bed hospital.[45] In setting up these hospitals, Christians were careful not to be associated with Greek and pagan philosophy, so, for example, the medical precepts of Hippocrates were discarded because of their pagan origins.

Monastic Hospitals

By the middle of the fourth century the founding and building of Christian hospitals were well under way. *Hospitia* was the original word for the way stations attached to monasteries that sheltered and fed tired travelers, pilgrims, refugees, and strangers and provided a place to cure the sick.[46] Hospitals were established in large cities in Asia Minor and in northern Mesopotamia.[47]

The hospitals and infirmaries were expressions of Christian charity and not for profit. This concept was entirely new in the pagan world. "The spirit of antiquity toward sickness and misfortune was not one of compassion," writes H. Fielding Garrison in his *History of Medicine*, "and the credit of ministering to human suffering on an extended scale belongs to Christianity."[48] With the fall of the Roman Empire the monasteries became the "centers" for social services that the state could no longer give.[49]

The Benedictines in the sixth century, and later the Franciscans in the thirteenth century, helped the poor and sick as a central part of their mission.[50] In England, the earliest hospital was built at St. Albans in 794 C.E. St. Thomas's Hospital is the continuation of a monastic charity of the thirteenth century, and St. Bartholomew's Hospital is of even earlier monastic origin.

Since leprosy was one of the Middle Ages' biggest killers—second only to the plague—one can understand why 200 of the 750 monastic hospitals in medieval England were for the care of people with leprosy.[51] The persistence of pestilence rather than the numbers of those wounded in wars contributed to the acceleration of the hospital movement, but both types of patients were treated. In addition to the emergency shelters that multiplied along the routes to nurse sick Crusaders, a two-thousand-bed military hospital was established in Palestine by the Order of St. John in 1099 C.E.[52] The purpose of hospitals such as St. Bartholomew's, founded in London in 1137 C.E., St. Thomas's, founded in 1207 C.E., and St. Mary of Bethlehem, founded in 1247 C.E., was to care for the sick.[53]

In the early Middle Ages almost all European medical practitioners were monks. However, by the thirteenth century this dual role was condemned for two reasons: (1) clerics used medicine as a way to earn money instead of performing it gratis; and (2) many people died, especially if surgery was involved, because of the monks' limited skills.[54] The rules of both St. Augustine and St. Benedict provided for a specific person, that is, an infirmarian, who was set apart to care for the sick so that the whole monastic community was not involved. Hence we have two contradictory phenomena, the official church losing interest in God's power to heal and individual Christians caring for the sick.

Transition from the Sacrament of Healing to Extreme Unction

It is generally agreed that a change in the understanding of unction occurred in the eighth and ninth centuries. Some attributed this change to the separation of sin and sickness and the church's interest in salvation rather than health. In other words, the sacrament of penance was originally for the confession of sins, but later confession also became part of extreme unction, making it a sacrament in its own right. Unction at that time focused on the remission of sins as its principal benefit and was regarded as a sacrament of the dying because of its association with deathbed penance. The majority of Anglican scholars believe that the James passage does not support the late medieval theory that unction was primarily ordained for the remission of sins; rather, they believe that it was for the healing of the whole person.[55]

During the Carolingian Renaissance in the ninth century, the sacrament became more clearly defined as its application narrowed. The first change was that the emphasis was more on the sacrament itself and less on the consecration of the oil; only priests, not laypeople, could anoint; the oil could be consecrated only by the bishop; and the sacrament became strongly affiliated with a penitential rite and with nearness of death. Since penance became increasingly severe—for example, starvation diets and abstention from marital intercourse—it is no wonder people preferred to wait until the end of their lives to perform their penances. The sacrament of healing became that of extreme unction; because it carried with it the forgiveness of sins, people postponed it to a point very near death. This change did not grow out of new theological insights into the meaning of the sacrament; it was the result of the historical situation of the people.[56]

During this period, the healing ministry was replaced by elaborate rites for the dying. They consisted of five parts: (1) visitation of the sick with the priest and family gathered around the bed in prayer; (2) confession of sin and absolution; (3) sacrament of extreme unction; (4) the last Holy Communion, that is, food for the journey (*viaticum*); and (5) the watch with the dying person and the commendation of the departing soul.

By the high Middle Ages (1050–1300 C.E.) the power of the Roman Catholic Church was based on moral coercion and social contract. The church offered a way for harmony with God while the peasants yearned for temporal well-being. The church condemned many of the superstitious practices of healing based on pagan rites, for example, the placing of a child on a roof or in an oven to cure a fever.[57] Prayer was a source of hope but lacked the glamour and efficacy of saints and relics that many Christians preferred.[58]

The emphasis on repentance of the sick person was based on Roman Catholic theology equating sin and sickness. Benefit was seen to derive from sickness, that is, it developed the virtue of patience. For example, when insanity led to suicide, causality was asserted though there was some ambiguity about drawing a direct correlation. In 1023 C.E. Fulbert of Chartres said, "It is a physician's duty to offer those who are suffering from depression, insanity, or any other illness what he has learned in the exercise of his art and to apply himself with all diligence to the task of curing them even if they are ungrateful and insult his skill."[59] Although the plague was seen as God's punishment, it was not necessarily assumed to be a punishment for a particular person's wrongdoing.[60]

In the later Middle Ages, Thomastic theology, which emphasized a hierarchy of soul, mind, and body, destroyed the sense of the unity of human nature that had hitherto existed. There occurred a divorce between salvation and health. Thomistic theology was influenced by Aristotle's closed view of the universe where the transcendent and healing miracles did not belong. "Religious experiences, however much they are part of the gospel proclamation, are excluded because they inconveniently do not fit into the pattern of logic and coherence that is at the heart of theological method."[61] Duns Scotus and Thomas Aquinas were the main interpreters of anointing as the removal of the last vestiges of sin, hence "extreme" unction. Aquinas taught that extreme unction was to prepare one for immediate entrance into heaven.[62] Thus, this sacrament was instituted principally for healing the sickness of sin. It is by grace that this sin is removed in immediate preparation for the beatific vision.

The Council of Trent

By the Council of Trent in 1551 the church regarded the needs of the soul in conflict with those of the body, and the gulf between science and religion, hence medicine and the church, widened.[63] Some scholars concluded from this that the true healing ministry of the church went underground and did not emerge again until the nineteenth century. The centrality of the sacraments continued, but the total spiritualization of unction reflected the disinterest in the body. The *Rituale Romanun* (1614) was for those in danger of death from sickness or old age. Unction then became preparation for death since the remission of sins was a central part of it.[64] "Our Redeemer . . . provided the greatest aids by means of which Christians may during life keep themselves free from every graver spiritual evil, so did He fortify the end of life by the sacrament of extreme unction as with the strongest defense."[65] Originally, anointing was "a sacrament of power for help to live," and later it became "a sacrament of authority to assure the passing [of the] soul."[66] The practice of extreme unction became part of a ceremony involving confession, absolution, viaticum, and anointing. This classical form of the sacrament was a preparation for the final judgment and was not changed until Vatican II (1962–65). However, the Council of Trent did not canonize the interpretation of extreme unction as solely a rite for the dying. The synod declared "that this anointing is to be applied to the sick, but especially to those who are in such danger as to appear to be at the end of life."[67]

In commenting on this sacrament, the Council of Trent stated that it is expedient not only for the health of the soul, but also to restore the health of the body. Overall, the council adapted the spiritual sense of *sozo* rather than the physical sense, though bodily health might result from strengthening of the soul.[68]

REFORMATION PERIOD—SEPARATION OF MEDICINE AND RELIGION AND REJECTION OF EXTREME UNCTION

Two factors influenced the Reformed churches' view of the ministry of healing: the rejection of many Roman Catholic practices and the increasing separation of medicine and religion.

The Protestant reformers' perspective on extreme unction was in sharp contrast to that of the Roman Catholic Church. The reformers associated anointing and laying on of hands with the Roman Catholic Church's practice of the sacrament of extreme unction. Since the reformers wished to separate themselves from many of Rome's practices, the rite fell into disuse. John Calvin (1509–64), the Swiss reformer, in his *Institutes* regards healing as a charismatic gift belonging to apostolic times and no longer applicable. Martin Luther (1483–1546) did not name unction as one of the sacraments but accepted the practice of anointing.

Luther and Calvin did not believe in miraculous physical healing but continued the medieval teaching of sickness as a chastisement or an occasion for moral teaching and death as an opportunity for release from the suffering of this world. Calvin wrote, "The heavenly physician treats some more gently but cleanses others by harsher remedies."[69] Calvin recognized creation as good but emphasized some separation between body and spirit.[70] He believed that suffering and sickness were not caused directly by God or by individual sin but by the breaking of the covenant in ways such as idol making and self-interest. Prayer and the forgiveness of sin could ease bodily sickness, and temperance as the basic approach to life was central for good health. Health was achieved within the Christian community by means of the body of Christ and by hearing and receiving God's Word. Calvin's contemporary, John Knox (ca. 1513–72), referred to Holy Communion as "singular medicine for the sick."[71]

Although they tended toward a spiritualized view of health, the reformers respected the medical profession. Calvin honored those who studied medicine, and it was not uncommon for reformers such as Richard Baxter (1615–91 C.E.) to dispense medical advice. Baxter's interest in health and sickness figures significantly in his practical works where he instructed the sick how to benefit from their illness by looking to their eternal salvation.[72] He urged Christians to follow physicians' advice rather than that of ignorant but well-meaning friends: "Use the best means for the recovery of the sick, which the ablest physicians shall advise you, as far as you are able."[73] Baxter further instructed ministers to preach to the sick and dying, capturing the reformed view that clergy could best comfort the sick through the Word.[74]

Like the reformers, the Church of England moved away from the practice of extreme unction. Anointing for healing made a brief appearance in the Anglican Church's 1549 Visitation of the Sick[75] only to disappear again because the provision in James 5 was not thought to be applicable.[76] The rite of anointing was deleted from the 1552 Anglican Prayer Book, but in the eighteenth and nineteenth centuries' reform movements, anointing was revived and is now firmly a part of Anglican practices. In the 1662 Prayer Book, the emphasis was on the need for repentance and confession since illness was seen as a matter of God's correction and for the building of faith and patience.[77] The sick were almost left with an obligation to die.

As products of the Enlightenment, Descartes (1596–1650 C.E.) and Newton (1642–1727 C.E.) had developed a mechanistic, dualistic view where spirit and matter were completely separated and determinism of the physical world was accepted. With a professionalization of ministry and medicine, the new practitioners, whose skills were "still primitive" by modern standards, had plenty of health problems to address, especially considering the high mortality rate of the times.[78]

Following the division of the church after the Reformation, there was also a growing split between religion and medicine. Phyllis Garlick draws the provocative parallel between the ecclesial fissure and "the new dawn of scientific medicine," which gave rise to "specialized classes of physicians and surgeons" during the Renaissance.[79] Healing by the church fell into disuse as the church yielded healing to the medical profession. The two became independent professions; specialization was mandated for both in the Western church.

In addition to the medicine/religion split, the breakup of the monasteries as a result of the Reformation ultimately shattered the caring system for the sick. As monasteries were closed (destroyed) between 1525 and 1540 C.E., so the "hospitals" disappeared with them. The Reformed churches did not have the agencies for the work of healing in place.[80] Luther effectively cut off the funding for health care by questioning the medieval motive of "gaining merit" by contributing to health care coffers. But what the reformers had lost in funding health care, Protestantism gained in social reform by addressing the underlying questions of sickness and poverty.[81]

In the eighteenth century (1720–50 C.E.), a number of voluntary hospitals were set up in London and some of the outlying cities. However, on the whole the state and individual cities set up organized charities to continue operating the hospitals whose roots were in Christianity.[82] The line of demarcation between the church's care of the soul and science's responsibility for physical health was firmly drawn in the seventeenth and eighteenth centuries and continued into modern times.[83]

THE MEDICAL MISSIONARY
MOVEMENT—HEALING AND SAVING

In a discussion of the early medical missionary movement, recognizing on the one hand the sacrificial contribution of the early doctors is important, while acknowledging on the other hand their rejection of most indigenous healing practices and their reliance on the medical model. To appreciate the rise of medical missions, we need to understand their spiritual roots in eighteenth-century Wesleyan revivalism. The latter was inspired by humanism and the zeal of German Pietism. This theology stressed the innate worth of all human beings and the duty of Christians to therefore reach out to others in heartfelt service. It was "concerned with the redemption of the individual, not of society," Garlick notes. "Theirs was an intensity of passion for individual souls, . . . for the millions dying without the knowledge of God."[84] Such a fire fueled the Protestant medical missionary movement.

Whereas the Roman Catholic Church drew its missionaries from monasteries, the Protestant missionary societies were composed of both laypersons and clergy because of their theology of the priesthood of all believers. These societies increased rapidly at the turn of the twentieth century. The new missionary impulse coincided with the juncture in world affairs when the rise of the British Empire began in Africa, India, and China.

The missionary movement was the principal force that took Western medical care to Africa, the Near East, India, and China to tackle leprosy, cholera, tuberculosis, and the plague, among other dreaded diseases. "Neither Hinduism nor Islam had evolved any social service as an expression of their faith, and the (other) states saw no necessity to spend money on healing the sick."[85] Among the arsenal contained in the black bags carried by medical missionaries were "[vaccination], the scientific treatment of epidemic and endemic diseases, the use of anaesthetics, and the practice of aseptic surgery," all paving the way for "modern nursing and medical education."[86]

Perhaps even more important than the introduction of Western science in addressing ills may have been the missionary attitude of concern for the sick and unselfish service for others that transformed the way people in these countries looked at caring for the sick. (I witnessed this dedication firsthand among medical missionaries such as Donald Gordon who worked for more than forty years, and later his son, Alan, for more than thirty years, ministering to the neediest in Brazil.)

In the best sense, the medical missionary movement placed technical cures within the wider context of "abundant living." The missionaries sought "to link up the science with the *source* of fuller life, by bringing men and women into living touch with the creative source—the Lord and Giver of life."[87] According to Garlick, this scientific advance was not the only factor that led to the extension of medical missions: "[a] new spiritual awakening; a wider interpretation of the Christian message to include social and spiritual needs at home and overseas; [and] a world open to the Gospel as never before"[88] conspired to carry medical missions into the twentieth century.

Medical missionaries went to the areas where the need was greatest. The mission hospitals provided an atmosphere of love and spiritual quiet that was more than basic medical care but rather the Christian ethic of love in action. A tribute panel over a building erected to Dr. van Someren Taylor in Fukien, China, captured the essence of mission work: "Far-spreading knowledge and kindness."[89] The early missionaries in the first half of the nineteenth century, upon seeing the terrible conditions of people in foreign lands, recognized that "preaching without healing was a most inadequate way of interpreting the Gospel."[90] The early medical mission work was often done by Christian medical societies and later incorporated into church boards.

The United States took the lead in expanding medical missions during the first half of the twentieth century. The mission work included the founding of hospitals and the establishing of public health measures. Mission hospitals such as one in Hangchow, China, cared not only for the general population but also for those wounded during the war with Japan.

The medical mission work with children in the carpet-weaving industry at Kerman, Persia, provides an illustration of the church's maturity in seeking to address the underlying problems causing illness. Tending to the children who were suffering from deformities and rickets, the doctors also set out to radically change the conditions in the industry itself. Well-baby clinics and prenatal care were additional elements in the preventive approach for dealing with the terrible diseases confronting the peoples of China, Persia, India, and Africa. The medical mission work flourished in response to these needs.

The subject of medical missions, of course, is fraught with perils. If the healing ministry is conducted simply to bring people into the church, its inherent good is overshadowed by its being used as a means to an end. The words from the 1939 Christian Medical Society statement are still illuminating today: "Medical missions, therefore do not exist merely to secure an audience for the Gospel, nor are they only a philanthropic agency. While their object is ever to bring men and women into personal touch with Jesus Christ, and to inspire the indigenous church with true ideals of Christian life and service, they must have regard for their primary task, the care of the sick and the prevention of disease."[91] Nevertheless, mission hospitals did see evangelism as essential, and many Christian doctors became voluntary evangelists in the hospitals.

As the period of medical missions ended, there was a movement from mission to church, from curative to preventive medicine, and from individual to community health and wholeness.[92] Most mission hospitals now have been nationalized, and U.S. denominational hospitals have been secularized and privatized. The recent paradigm shift in the Two Thirds World is moving health care delivery from the hospital-based medical missionary movement model toward a more integrated health- and community-based model, empowering people to be responsible for their own health. The reasons for this shift are (1) the exorbitant cost of establishing and sustaining health institutions; (2) alternative sources of health care provided by government and private organizations in many countries; (3) the difficulty by a number of countries in managing large medical institutions that exceed local competency levels and specialties; and (4) the shift in North American missiology from building institutions to empowering and enabling people in preventive health care based on a wholistic, communitarian vision of health.[93]

Rather than building expensive hospitals, the church is trying to work with communities to address root problems such as water supply, hygiene, nutrition, and health education—things that improve people's standard of living. A great deal of money can be spent and resources used on doctors and nurses to treat diarrhea, or one can determine the root cause of diarrhea. The use of resources already available locally, such as indigenous healers, helps people to be in charge of their own health.

POSTMODERN RESISTANCE TO THE CHURCH'S HEALING MINISTRY

Since the waning of medical missions, from the 1950s until the 1980s, the healing ministry of the church has been neither fully successful nor very prominent due to a variety of factors: (1) the previously mentioned nationalization of mission hospitals and the change to community-based health care left the church without a familiar model for health ministries;[94] (2) unorthodox theological perspectives and the involvement of fringe healing groups drove this ministry to the margins of the church's mission; (3) the church had only the vaguest notion of concrete ways to integrate a healing ministry into its total life and mission; (4) the church lacked a firm educational basis for training physicians to develop a theological perspective on whole person medicine or for teaching pastors about primary health care, and it provided few or no opportunities for interchange between students and professionals on health issues; and (5) little verifiable data existed to persuade the scientific community of the church's effectiveness as a health care institution.

In recent decades, traditional denominations were often critical of parachurch and nondenominational groups engaged in healing ministries. When these groups tried to reproduce the New Testament and early church methods exclusively by anointing, laying on of hands, and casting out of demons, without acknowledging contemporary medical practices, they became marginalized. The effectiveness of these healing ministries is measured only by positive testimonials gathered in emotional moments, without recognizing those whose hopes were dashed and who suffered at the hands of these so-called healers.[95] Many impostors traded on the credulity of people and set themselves up as faith healers, ultimately driving some people away from the church. Since the process of cause and effect in Christian faith healing is not readily seen, allegiance was shifted to science.[96] Faith did not disappear, but was merely transferred from a piece of bone or shrine to a petri dish.

THE RISE OF A NEW DISCIPLINE—HEALTH MINISTRIES

Despite modern skepticism, a new movement is afloat that is dramatically changing society's and the church's view of the healing ministry. The ecumenical expansion of the healing ministry in new and creative ways is a sign of a real recovery of the church's historic role, not just the idiosyncratic work of a handful of pastors. Churches once again are taking seriously Christ's charge to heal as well as responding to the needs for compassionate care in the midst of the current marketplace medicine milieu. As was mentioned in the preface, this new discipline of health ministries has historic roots that represent the convergence of many streams. The conversation between medicine and religion, the growth of sacramental and charismatic healing ministries, the development of bioethics, medical missions work, wholistic health care practices, the acceptance of complementary health care practices, and, most recently, the popular interest in spirituality and health are the principal foundations for health ministries.

The British Context

In describing the current rise of the church's health ministry, it is helpful to look at both the British and the U.S. context. In the late 1970s and 1980s the churches in the United Kingdom were far ahead of those in the United States in developing a healing ministry. Denis Duncan, a British theologian, discusses this phenomenon and rightly points out that the healing ministry is not some new policy to respond to loss of members but part of the historical mission of the church.[97] The long history of a sacramental ministry in the Church of England provides a fertile ground for a healing ministry that is not as true in the United States. Therefore, the healing ministry initially developed in somewhat different forms in the United States.

The different sources of the current British health ministry are (1) the founding of the Guild of St. Raphael in 1915, which is distinctly Anglo-Catholic and sacramentalist with an emphasis on the ministry of the priest visiting the sick; (2) the development of the Guild of Health in 1904 and other healing agencies that were interested in psychology and healing services, and stressed a theology that health was God's will for us; and (3) the emergence of the charismatic movement in the 1960s with the practice of laying on of hands and the expectation that God would work miracles of physical healing.[98]

According to Charles Gusmer, a British theologian, additional factors that led to the emergence of the healing ministry in the Anglican Church were the discussion of this subject at the Lambeth Conferences from 1908, 1920, 1930, and 1958; the promulgation of official rites of healing by the Canterbury (1935) and York (1936) convocations; the founding of the Churches' Council for Health and Healing (CCHH) in the United Kingdom; a growing cooperation between clergy and the medical profession; the Report of the Archbishops' Commission on Healing in 1953; the founding of the Institute of Religion and Medicine in 1961, which grew out of a meeting of priests and doctors; and the beginning of various health guilds and organizations of healing such as the previously mentioned Guild of Health, the Guild of St. Raphael, and the Divine Healing Mission. These organizations worked in close harmony with doctors, advocating wholistic health, while lifting up the spiritual healing of the church.[99] From 1968 to 1993 a bimonthly journal, *The Way of Life*, was published jointly by the Guilds of Health and St. Raphael.

The Guild of St. Raphael emphasizes four features of the healing ministry—prayer and intercession, absolution, unction and laying on of hands, and Holy Communion. It has always emphasized cooperation with the medical profession.[100] The Divine Healing Mission was founded in 1905 by lay healer James Hickson, who received Archbishop Davidson's blessing to start a healing ministry. On Hickson's visit to Iona in 1917, God showed him the plan to take the message of the healing ministry around the world, which he did. He had a great impact in Ireland, Rome,

Paris, South Africa, and other places he visited concerning the importance of the healing ministry in the life of the church.[101] Meanwhile in 1912 Dorothy Kerin, who at age twenty-three was healed of tubercular peritonitis after months of being an invalid, began a healing ministry. This led to the founding of the Dorothy Kerin Trust, which eventually became a Home of Healing in Burrswood, England; religion and medicine are closely associated in this facility.

The Lambeth Conferences Discuss the Healing Ministry

As was previously mentioned, the Lambeth Conferences played an important role in the British healing ministry. The Lambeth Conference is convened about every ten years by the Anglican Church to discuss matters of doctrine and faith in the life of the church. The work of William Temple in the United Kingdom, especially in the 1920 Lambeth Conference, represented a landmark event by producing recommendations about the healing ministry for the Church of England. The report urged the whole communion to be involved in the ministry of healing by teaching about it, cooperating with the medical profession, and developing intercessory prayer groups in every parish.[102] Temple's initiatives eventually led to the formation of the Churches' Council for Health and Healing.

The committee members who prepared the documents for the Lambeth Conferences wrestled with various aspects of the healing ministry. In 1908 they were concerned with Christian Scientists whom they labeled as false healers.[103] The conference, however, addressed one of its principal concerns of sacramental healing functions. It did not specifically forbid or reinstitute the sacrament of healing but said if the sick persons wanted it, they could receive anointing with oil. However, the conference warned that it should not be administered as a preparation for death.

In 1924 Lambeth addressed the question of different methods of bodily healing, citing three types: (1) material (surgery, drugs, diet); (2) psychical (mental analysis); and (3) devotional and sacramental. "Spiritual healing," they said, can be used in all three of these areas if reliance on God is central. The conference specifically warned against equating spiritual healing with only the third method. However, primary emphasis was on the healing of the spirit, bodily healing being secondary. Patients should not look to the clergy to do what is the physician's duty.[104] The 1924 Lambeth Committee also recommended the ancient sequence of reconciliation, anointing, and communion for the rite of healing. Subsequent pastoral care was considered as important as the preparation with a period of tranquillity and peace after the rite. The pastor would offer thanksgiving with the patient the next day if possible. The revision of the service for "Ministry to the Sick" in the Anglican Church was much needed because of the outdated nature of the service of 1662, which left the sick person not only with the expectation of impending death, but almost a duty to die. The 1928 Deposited Book attempted to deal with both problems. The communion of the sick provided for permanent reservation of the consecrated elements to allow for their distribution to those not present. Since the practice was controversial, the 1928 Deposited Book was rejected because of this very issue.

In the 1930s, the Canterbury and York Convocations took separate action to provide forms for the laying on of hands with prayers for the sick as well as anointing. The status of such rites was ambiguous, and the Guild of St. Raphael's unofficial services were widely used. However, the service of anointing was reinstituted in the 1935 Book of Common Prayer. Geoffrey Harding wrote, "If baptism means renewal of life, anointing its restoration, and communion its continuing enjoyment, then anointing as it were looks backwards to baptism and forward to the Eucharist."[105] The belief was that the anointing of a baptized person in time of sickness may be a rehallowing of one whose body and spirit have been affected by sin. The patient was to prepare for anointing by penitence and faith; hence absolution was often linked with the administration of the rite. If the patient cannot respond, a prayer can be made on her behalf that expresses her desire for forgiveness. This rite should be practiced as part of the communion service. It may bring physical healing but, most important, enables one to grasp the "strong hand of our Deliverer and to pass peacefully and fearlessly with [God] through the valley."[106]

In the Revised Catechism of 1962 the church provides for other "'sacramental ministries of grace': confirmation, ordination, holy matrimony, the ministry of absolution and the ministry of healing."[107] "The sacramental ministry of healing is the ministry by which God's grace is given for the healing of spirit, mind and body, in response to faith and prayer, by the laying on of hands, or by anointing with oil."[108]

The thrust of the Lambeth Conferences in recent decades has been to urge the whole Anglican community to be involved in a ministry of healing. The 1988 conference emphasized the following purposes of the healing ministry: restoration of a sense of relationship with God and the community; affirmation of the body's natural healing powers; utilization of all medical knowledge and skills to cure, restore, or relieve pain; acceptance of both our mortality and our eternal destiny, which will foster inner peace. The healing ministry was understood to include medical research; the prevention of disease and the promotion of healthy lifestyles; the inclusion of the medical and caring professions; the ministries of prayer and the sacraments; and the counseling and support of all those who are troubled, sick, and dying.[109]

The 1988 Lambeth Conference went so far as to say that the ministry of healing should be established in every diocese. It should expand beyond sacramental ministries to include counseling, deliverance from demonic oppression, medical research, and the study of related ethical issues; it should work for fair distribution of resources and personnel; and it should include drug addicts, sufferers from AIDS, and the work of hospices. In addition, the archbishops of Canterbury and York in 1983 appointed Bishop Morris Maddocks as their advisor on health and healing, thereby underscoring the church's dedication to health ministry. Maddocks has written a number of books on health ministry as well as setting up the Acorn Christian Healing Trust. (The Acorn Trust is a team of teachers, enablers, and pastors who now travel the world as well as a resource and conference center for seminars on the church's healing ministry in Hampshire, England.[110])

The most noteworthy group carrying forward the healing ministry is the previously mentioned Churches' Council for Health and Healing (CCHH), which embraces all the major denominations in the United Kingdom along with the principal medical bodies such as the Royal College of Physicians. It began as an umbrella organization for all healing ministries in Britain, but the numbers became so vast that it could no longer claim to embrace them all. (It disbanded in 1999, with hopes of forming a successor group.) In 1947 the British Medical Association (BMA) issued a statement welcoming the existence of the CCHH: "Medicine and the Church working together should encourage a dynamic philosophy of health which would enable every citizen to find a way of life based on moral principles and on a sound knowledge of the factors which promote health and well-being. Health is more than a physical problem, and the patient's attitude both to illness and to other problems is an important factor to his recovery and adjustment to life." Interestingly enough, as strong a support as this is, the BMA found no evidence of illness healed by spiritual healing alone but admitted to the psychological value of sound religious ministrations and encouraged cooperation between clergy and physicians.[111] This attitude, however, can foster a dualistic approach where the doctor handles the body and the church handles the soul.

Ecumenical Healing Ministry in Great Britain

Morris Maddocks credits much of the British Methodist Church's interest in healing to Leslie Weatherhead, Methodist preacher and author, especially to his classic work, *Psychology, Religion, and Healing*, written in 1951. Weatherhead wrote extensively on the phenomenon of healing, including his discussion of "odic" force.[112] The Methodists now have a healing and pastoral ministry committee as part of their Division of Social Responsibility and continue to emphasize the healing ministry.[113]

Other denominations such as the United Reformed Church formed a health committee, which produced the study kit "Health and Healing" in 1977 with instructions for sacramental healing. In addition, the Rev. David Dale, moderator of the General Assembly of the United Reformed Church in the 1980s, and the Rev. Howard Booth in the Methodist Church provided strong leadership in this area. The Baptist Union formed a committee on health and healing. The Roman Catholic Church reinstituted its ministry of healing at the Second Vatican Council, returning extreme unction to the sacrament of healing, which is practiced in Roman Catholic churches throughout the United Kingdom.[114]

Maddocks goes on to cite a number of Americans in the last two centuries whose healing ministries had an impact in the United Kingdom: A. J. Gordon, the famous Baptist minister in Boston, wrote a book on healing in 1882, and Elwood Worcester began his ministry in 1905 at Cgyrcg/Ennabyek. Then beginning in the 1950s, Agnes Sanford's, Kathryn Kuhlman's, and Oral Roberts's healing ministries had a large following in the United Kingdom. Interestingly enough, many of those who wrote about and practiced a healing ministry were not clergy in mainline denominations but worked freelance or in parachurch groups. An exception was Francis MacNutt, a Roman Catholic priest who was part of the Catholic charismatic movement.

Healing ministries currently practiced in the United Kingdom include the laying on of hands, anointing, prayer, and healing services. Sometimes a single clergy, a team of healers, or church members conduct the healing ministry. Healing ministries have become so popular because people believe spiritual healing works; how and why are not of concern. Stephen Pattison, a British pastoral theologian and consultant, believes one reason for the boom in health ministries is a sectarianism that emphasizes sacramentalism and other distinct practices. This, of course, refers to the Anglican Church's focus on the sacraments as vehicles for healing. Further popularity of healing ministries comes in light of a growing secularism where the healing ministry reaffirms the unique function of the church. Pattison cautions, however, that such a focus can cause abuse of the church's "power."[115] In addition, there is a renewed interest in spirituality, art, and medicine in medical practices such as that of Malcolm Rigler in Birmingham and the one at Bromley by Bow in East London.

Religion/Medicine Interface
Lays Foundation for Health Ministries

One interesting way of understanding both the U.S. and the U.K. development of this new discipline of health ministries is to look more closely at the history of the interface between religion and medicine. This relationship has been either adversarial or indifferent. In England until the end of the seventeenth century, physicians and other medical practitioners were licensed by diocesan bishops. In seventeenth- and eighteenth-century England there was considerable overlap between medical and religious professionals. By the mid-nineteenth century, because of the Medical Registration Act, all but qualified doctors were excluded from practicing medicine, so religion and health care were formally separated.

The development of the Protestant church's concern for a health ministry stems in part from John Wesley who, as previously mentioned, also influenced the development of medical missions. In the early eighteenth century he combined a spiritual evangelism with a social gospel rooted in the people's needs including their health care. Health was of great concern considering that England recorded the highest death rate in its history at that time.[116]

Wesley was one of the principal pastor/theologians to note the integral relationship between religion and health. He understood that health care was connected with lifestyle. In 1746 he founded the first free medical dispensary in England. His *Primitive Physic*[117] was a book full of practical advice about diet, exercise, sleep, and other basic elements of self-care. The founder of Methodism believed the love of God helped to keep the passions in their due bounds. Tranquillity could contribute to health and long life. "It is no mere accident that the most marked increase in the standard of public health coincided with the growing influence of the revival movement."[118] By leading the way for helping the suffering poor who had been neglected by the medical profession, Wesley became a pioneer of the national health movement. Can the same be said for the church today?

Unfortunately, other denominations did not adopt Wesley's insights. During the next hundred years with the increase of scientific knowledge about health and disease, a more materialistic and mechanistic view of life gradually dominated. The church often clung to outdated theories about the nature of illness. In many ways, the church was the principal cause of the separation of medicine and religion. For example, James Young Simpson's discovery of the use of chloroform as an anesthesia met with strong opposition from the church. "By bringing children into the world without pain, Simpson was accused of flying in the face of Providence, for had not God said that man should be born in pain? To which Simpson, himself skilled in theological argument, retorted that when God made Eve out of Adam's rib God first caused Adam to fall into a deep sleep which showed that God, the Creator, appreciated anaesthesia."[119] Three of the greatest medical discoverers—Louis Pasteur, James Young Simpson, and Joseph Lister—were men of deep religious faith. However, the history of the relationship between medicine and religion seems to be basically one of conflict.[120]

Moving from the post-Reformation and Enlightenment into modern times, there was an attempt to reintegrate salvation and health, broadening health from an individual to a community concern. As previously noted, during the nineteenth and twentieth centuries the church's establishment of hospitals worldwide strengthened in new ways its healing ministry. However, the church principally followed the medical model of sickness rather than that of preventive health care.

In the nineteenth century those of the Reformed faith emphasized public health measures and certain standards of living and lifestyles as producing good health. The professionalization of both ministry and medicine that had resulted in the rift between them yielded in the 1960s and 1970s to a strong cooperation. A number of professional societies were established to encourage the interaction between medicine and religion. In the 1960s and 1970s in the United Kingdom there was the establishment of clergy-doctor associations such as the previously mentioned Institute of Religion and Medicine. Physicians such as Robert Lambourne and Michael Wilson and clergy such as Michael Melinsky provided a rationale and model for the cooperation between mainstream Christianity and modern medicine.

At the same time, ecumenical bodies such as the National Council of Churches, American Protestant denominational headquarters, and Catholic organizations set up numerous programs and organizations to foster this cooperation. Health as a social justice issue was emphasized in organizations such as the Christian Medical Commission of the World Council of Churches, which introduced community-based health care as essential and provided an international network of those interested in wholistic health.

However, these cooperative endeavors between medicine and religion declined in the late 1970s and 1980s. For example, the membership of the Institute of Religion and Medicine in 1983 was half of what it was in 1971. The institute, which disbanded in 1993, was incorporated into the Churches' Council for Health and Healing and was known as the Medical Forum; it had a membership of two hundred. British clergy, on the whole, according to Pattison and others, find little interest among doctors for working cooperatively.[121] Two reasons may be that the early groups were essentially homogeneous and local clergy still operated within the purely sacramental and spiritual models. In the United States the former Society for Health and Human Values founded in the 1970s by a physician, Edmund Pellegrino, and a Presbyterian higher education staff person, Ron McNuer, gradually absorbed a more diverse constituency and lost its principal focus on clergy-physician dialogue. In addition, the whole field of bioethics, which initially grew out of ethical and religious questions, moved away from theology to philosophy and medicine for its grounding.[122]

The Expansion of Health Ministries in the United States

The factors that have influenced the exponential growth of health ministries in the United States are (1) concern about universal access to health care (44 million people are without health insurance), especially the exclusion of immigrants and certain racial/ethnic groups, loss of health care insurance by the unemployed, and rising out-of-pocket costs for medical care; (2) criticisms of the medical model (Ivan Illich and others have exposed the "iatrogenesis" where doctors may cause more harm than good; even avoiding extremists like Illich, numerous critics of the medical model make clergy and patients alike wary);[123] (3) establishment of various organizations that work at the interface of medicine and religion, for example, the American Society for Bioethics and Humanities (formerly Society for Health and Human Values), Park Ridge Center, bioethics institutes such as the Kennedy Institute of Ethics at Georgetown University, Hastings Center, and hundreds of others; (4) church-linked health-related programs such as Alcoholics Anonymous and other twelve-step groups; Meals-on-Wheels, respite care programs, day care centers, and exercise classes that use church buildings; and (5) African American churches that sponsor social programs such as shelter and meal programs, employment assistance, tutoring, blood pressure control, and so forth, which stem from a real need in light of their segregation and marginalization from many of society's programs. These various factors have opened the way for new avenues of church involvement in health issues.

In the 1970s there were hundreds of groups, now there are thousands, engaging in health ministries. In the United Kingdom, reference is made to the healing ministry; in the United States, it is to health ministry programs. This highlights the distinction between the Anglican Church's emphasis on sacramental and spiritual healing as historically practiced versus the programmatic emphasis of U.S. churches on education and direct health care services.

The new openness to holistic health by health care professionals may also help to legitimize the healing ministry of the church. Some believe that the current acceptance of holistic health is due to an openness among the medical professions to take into account psychosomatic factors in illness.[124] However, it is questionable if the move from psychosomatic to spiritual healing is an automatic one. Freudian psychology embraced the medical model and accepted the psychosomatic dimension of illness. But it shunned and strongly criticized religion as being detrimental to our mental health rather than enhancing it. The resurgence of interest in spirituality may reflect a deep hunger for the transcendent and a search for a deeper purpose in the face of the materialism of our age. This interest, though, does not necessarily link to an acceptance of the church's role in health.

The recent interest in the renewal of Christian healing may be attributable to the change from the compartmentalization of physics, medicine, biology, politics, and ecology to a more holistic approach. It recognizes the intricate interrelationship between emotions, body, and mind; the challenge to rationalism by the embracing of the transcendent and spiritual; and the openness of many people to the Holy Spirit, which gives power for healing ministries.[125] There is a greater opportunity for cooperation with medicine than ever before; we should refer to the healing ministry of the church not as an alternative therapy but as a complementary one.

Another sign of the expansion of health ministries is the introduction of healing and prayer services into the general worship life of the church of most Protestant denominations. Presbyterians, Lutherans, Episcopalians, Mennonites, and Baptists, among others, hold frequent healing services; ten years ago that would not have been the case. Liturgies of healing are now included in several denominational supplementary worship books.

Many of the health ministries programs focus on direct health care and prevention including collaborative programs with community agencies, not just liturgical aspects of health ministry. In addition, networks of physicians and clergy in the mainstream of the church and medicine have been developing cooperative health care delivery systems. The Park Ridge Center in Chicago is analyzing the interface between medicine and religion; churches in the 1980s in Massachusetts created a network of Wellness Centers. The Wholistic Health Centers, Inc. (WHC) and parish nurse programs, established by Granger Westberg, provide evidence of the effectiveness of church-based, whole person health care.[126] A Kellogg Foundation study covering an eleven-year period showed that in Chicago, WHC patients had one-fifth the hospitalization days in comparison to the average for other patients. According to the International Parish Nurse Resource Center, the parish nurse program, which began in the early

1980s with a few dozen nurses serving as ministerial staff linking the hospital and the church, has expanded to several thousand parish nurses in the late 1990s. At least monthly, articles cite newly established parish nurse programs around the country.

The 1992 National Council of Churches' survey of congregations, representing sixteen Protestant denominations, showed that 78 percent of them are addressing at least one health concern while half are addressing three or more.[127] Mental health, nutrition, substance abuse, access to medical care, immunization, and health insurance coverage are only a few of the issues that these churches are addressing in health care.

The Health Ministries Association, founded in 1989 with a few dozen members, now has 1,100 members throughout the United States and in several other countries. Its membership grows weekly as new churches begin health ministries programs; it recently voted to become interfaith in its thrust, which reflects the growing interest in religion and health.

In light of this rich history of the church's involvement in health and healing, the question is, What will the twenty-first century bring? What will be our response to the frail, lonely elderly persons whose medical insurance has run out? Or the illegal aliens, who dare not seek any medical help whatsoever? Will we consider homeless people, whose life expectancy is probably half that of the average white male? It is as we respond to the health needs in our own backyard that we as a church show something of the character of God. In the following chapters we will examine new areas of health ministry programs and initiatives.

2

The Fullness of Time for a New Health Ministry

As was noted at the end of the last chapter, new forms of the church's healing ministry, that is, health ministry, have emerged. There are a variety of reasons why the church's health ministry is coming to bloom. They stem not only from the changing face of illness and the breakdown of traditional health care systems but also from the acceptance of more holistic health care practices and the scientific verification of the positive role of religious beliefs, practices, and worshiping communities. Understanding these factors forms the basis for developing effective and needed programs so the church can return to its rightful place as a major health care provider.

THE CHANGING NATURE OF ILLNESS

The first reason this is the fullness of time for the church's health ministry is the changing nature of illness. We are healthier today than ever before. (In 1996, the average life expectancy for North American white females was 79.6 years and black females 74.2; white males 73.8 years and black males 66.1; and all nonwhite population 71.9 years;[1] in 1997, the life expectancy for females and males in Great Britain was 79.9 and 74.6, respectively).[2] Many doctors claim that our longevity has more to do with changes in diet and sanitation than with scientific medicine. Furthermore, the face of illness has changed in these past decades with lifestyle diseases—that is, alcohol-related car accidents, suicide, and homicide—the leading killers of teenagers and young adults up to twenty-five years of age.

Violent crimes are now listed as health problems by the U.S. Centers for Disease Control. Two out of every three deaths in the United States are premature or unnecessary. Chronic conditions are the major causes of illness, disability, and death in the United States today. The increase in the survival of newborns with genetic anomalies and chronic conditions, and a larger aging population have increased the number of disabilities attributable to long-term illness and congenital abnormalities.[3] Acute disease resulting in an early death has drastically declined due to antimicrobial and anti-infective drugs. Society focuses increasingly on function and quality of life now that the problem of longevity, in a relative sense, has been solved.[4]

Scientific medicine alone is not sufficient to address these new illnesses. Medical care affects only 10 percent of the indices used to measure health status.[5] The microbiologist and experimental pathologist René Dubos believed that life expectancy increased more as a result of reduced infant mortality, better nutrition, and sanitary practices than from drugs or medical treatment.[6]

The discussions of lifestyle, socioeconomic class, and injustice against certain classes and races of people as contributing to health and sickness provide secular versions of the biblical perspective that both our external and our internal worlds affect our health. *Health, United States, 1998* "includes a special study of socioeconomic disparities in health. For almost all health indicators considered, each increase in either income or education increased the likelihood of being in good health."[7] Stress factors such as tension, fear, anxiety, apprehension, and mistrust create a disunity that produces illness of mind and body.[8] "Marital status, income, and education may affect health characteristics in several ways. Higher income and education may provide family members with more knowledge of good health habits and better access to health and preventive services. Persons living with a spouse are likely to have better health profiles because of lifestyle differences (such as better eating habits, someone to share a problem) and higher incomes."[9]

THE CRISIS IN HEALTH CARE

The current crisis in health care offers the church a unique opportunity to reclaim its place in the health care arena. The shortcomings of the current medical model, the failure of health care reform, and the disenchantment with managed care have created a void that the church is qualified to fill.[10]

Not only are we experiencing a crisis in the United States, but the National Health Service in the United Kingdom is breaking down with shrinking funds, the expansion of parallel private services, and the transition to doctors as fund holders.[11] In the United States the failure of systematic health care reform, the difficulties with managed care, and the continual rise of health care costs offer an opportunity for new health care partners. Because of the disenchantment with managed care, or as some refer to it, managed cost, the church can serve as a central partner in the provision of health care if it provides ways to reduce cost while expanding care. Religious communities are being viewed as new collaborators, forming the basis for the unique role of the church in addressing lifestyle-related illnesses.

There are fundamental economic reasons for broadening traditional medical practice to include the church as a provider. In response to the high cost of health care, the U.S. Department of Health and Human Services, private health care groups, and industry are beginning to emphasize sickness prevention. The church has sponsored numerous effective health care programs, which are discussed in chapter 10. Wellness courses offered by churches are supplementing preventive medicine initiatives of health maintenance organizations (HMOs) and preventive care institutes; compliance with healthy practices in church-based health education programs is much higher than in community-based programs. In addition, the use of church buildings for primary health care clinics can reduce the health care costs associated with new construction.

EXPANSION OF HEALTH CARE PRACTICES

The emergence of complementary health care practices has also made this the fullness of time for the church's health ministry. Various means for healing may be used by the patient, family, friends, church members, and traditional health care professionals. They include physical methods such as diet, adequate sleep, exercise, clean water, and adequate housing; medical means such as surgery, drugs, tests, and treatments; emotional factors such as affection, touch, compassion, presence of friends and family, support groups, and self-help groups; spiritual resources such as the offering of hope, prayer, and worship, faith of friends and the patient; and psychological means of counseling, therapy, and imaging. As we embrace a more wholistic vision of healing, all resources can be means of God's healing grace while we cooperate with the God-given process of healing. The church then becomes a natural partner in health care.

It is true, however, that these broader practices for healing may promise more than they can deliver. They may feed into the U.S. aspiration for perfection, a utopianism that eventually disappoints. Realism argues for the tempering of expectations. Once expectations are tempered, the patient may come to appreciate that while complete healing may not be possible, some healing is always available—deterrents to health can be removed. What are the deterrents that need to be eliminated? Or put positively, what factors contribute to health? These factors include genetic (what we have received through our parents); physiological (how the body has developed); sociological (our natural and human environment); economic (class, income); lifestyle (job, marital status, diet, exercise); philosophical/theological (value system and religious beliefs); and psychological (self-esteem, integration of the personality). Verifiable data in the last several decades about the importance of most of these factors in contributing to health have led to their general acceptance by the medical profession.

Recognition of Psychosomatic Illness Broadened Healing Practices

The first dent in the armor of strictly scientific medicine's dominance was the acceptance of psychosomatic medicine from the 1950s onward. It is now commonly practiced but initially was challenged by the scientific community until corroborating data could be produced to prove the mind-body effect. The increased studies and literature that substantiate the mind-body interaction have made it more widely accepted. Ken Pelletier, clinical associate professor of medicine at Stanford University School of Medicine, claims that all four major categories of disease in the United States—cardiovascular, cancer, arthritis, and respiratory disorders—are increasingly seen as psychosomatic.[12] Even accidents may be cries for help and attention. Nikolas Tinbaergen, 1973 Nobel Prize winner for physiology and medicine, observed, "The more we discover about psychosomatic diseases and the extremely complex two-way traffic between the brain and the rest of the body, it is obvious that the too-rigid distinction between mind and body limits the advance of medical science."[13]

The broadening of the mind-body model to the bio-psycho-social one of George Engel and others may bring wider acceptance of the interaction of the *spirit* with the body, broadening our model of healing. Many cases and stories are told of the spirit's power to heal or injure, and scientific data are being gathered to corroborate this phenomenon. From psychosomatic medicine we now move to the more recent acceptance of nonallopathic health care practices, that is, those not based solely on scientific medicine.

Nonallopathic Healing Practices Defined

What we are witnessing today is a dramatic shift from strict adherence to the medical model or allopathic medicine, which has controlled health care in this country for the past several decades. Health care professionals from diverse backgrounds are advocating the expansion of health care to include more than the scientific, medical treatment of organic diseases. In part, this perspective is reflected in the whole person medicine approach to health care that is appearing in some medical school curricula.

Defining various nonallopathic practices is important since terms such as "traditional," "alternative," and "spiritual healing" are used in confusing and fuzzy ways. What the United States calls alternative medicine is traditional medicine for 80 percent of the world, and what the United States calls traditional medicine, that is, scientific medicine, is only a few centuries old. When the two are wedded, they form what is known as integrative or complementary medicine.[14] To understand complementary medicine, we will examine folkloric, alternative, holistic, and nonallopathic health care practices; these represent an East-West blend of medicine. Indigenous healing practices are often culture specific, and alternative medicine may embrace acupuncture, psychic healing, therapeutic touch, yoga, and a variety of related techniques. Other writers refer to building medical systems at the household level. These ethnomedical systems represent a blend of the medical model—traditional and home remedies passed from one generation to another.[15] Health care delivery systems that recognize and embrace these alternative approaches with acceptance of value-matched systems can improve health care.[16]

Contrast between Wholistic and Holistic

The emergence of these new healing practices also brings with them a new vocabulary that requires such fine linguistic distinctions as those between wholistic and holistic health care. Wholistic health care, promoted by Granger Westberg (retired hospital chaplain and founder of the Wholistic Health Centers and parish nursing), is rooted in a Christian perspective of integrated health care of mind, body, and spirit with God as the source of all healing. Holistic health care, on the other hand, represents the international movement spearheaded by Andrew Weil, the Harvard-educated physician who has appeared in *Life, Newsweek*, and other magazines as the guru of New Age health practices. It embraces a wide variety of traditional and alternative health care practices, where spirit is interpreted from an

Eastern religious perspective and exotic practices are included that blend alternative and allopathic approaches.

Guided by practitioners such as Weil, alternative and holistic medicine become synonymous. Weil refers to the lunar and solar aspects of the human mind. He has studied the firewalkers in Asian countries and the sweat lodges of American Indians where practitioners survive extreme heat without ill effects. These seeming miracles come from group concentration to bring about a desired result.[17] Weil asserts that his professional life has been devoted to the philosophy of "Patient, heal thyself." As reflected in his book *Spontaneous Healing*, his prescription includes deep yogic breathing, eating garlic, buying fresh flowers, and being with friends who make you laugh, although he also gives the more conventional advice of regular exercise, eating well, avoiding unnecessary toxins, and doing volunteer work.[18] He states, "My gut estimate is that conventional medicine is appropriate for about 15 to 20 percent of the instances in which we're now using it. If we restricted it to those instances, we wouldn't have an economic crisis in health care."[19] He does not eliminate but limits the uses of allopathic medicine. Weil, in many ways, is the prime leader of holistic health. His Web site in April 1997 alone had one million hits.[20]

The holistic movement, especially in health care, challenges the long-held grounding of medicine in a kind of materialism. This materialism operated from a mechanistic model of the human organism. The holistic view of medicine by contrast operates from a unitive understanding of materialism and spirituality, and it is beginning to receive a serious hearing with the Alternative Medicine Institute at the National Institutes of Health (NIH) started in 1992 and in the United Kingdom with the British Holistic Medical Association (BHMA). It is fascinating to read the principles of the BHMA published in 1984, which refer to the human organism as multidimensional, possessing body, mind, and spirit, interconnected to our environment, and innately capable of healing ourselves.

Alternative (Complementary) Health Care Practices Gain Acceptance

As was suggested when discussing the holistic movement, alternative medicine is broadly defined by its practitioners. The most definitive guide to date, produced by the National Institutes of Health, includes a discussion of a wide range of alternative medicine practices.[21] Alternative medicine, according to some such as Robert C. Fuller, professor of philosophy and religious studies at Bradley University, has a symbiotic relationship with the nineteenth-century antielitism flavor of Jacksonian Americans, who criticized the monopoly of professionals.[22] This perspective created the climate for homeopathic medicine so widely practiced in Europe and now growing in the United States. Fred M. Frohock writes, "Followers of allopathic and holistic medicine do not simply see the world differently; they see different worlds."[23] For some, it consists of Eastern practices such as yoga, massage, acupuncture, and more than thirty techniques including "cupping" (ancient practice to improve circulation) and rolfing.[24] Chiropractic, herbal and vitamin therapies, meditation, and therapeutic touch are also examples of alternative medicine. Some embrace New Age approaches such as crystals and channeling as part of alternative health care, and still others include spiritual and religious practices under alternative medicine. Described as an art rather than a science,[25] alternative medicine seeks to treat the individual "as a unity of body, mind and soul. An individual's biological makeup and his or her personality and spiritual orientation are deemed critical" to the person's illness, healing, and growth.[26] Patients claim to be treated more as partners than consumers and as sick people searching for health rather than depersonalized illnesses.

In alternative medicine, the three communities of allopathic medicine, psychology, and religion merge. Medical doctors, psychotherapists, theologians, and clergy become equal partners in the healing process. But while alternative medicine includes traditional medical treatment in the hospital setting as an option within its definition, allopathic medicine does not so embrace this holistic approach. Most people prefer the term "complementary" medicine to "alternative." Here the word "medicine" is deleted altogether, given its allopathic association, and instead the term "complementary health care" is used. Furthermore, I would argue that the four categories of health ministries later presented could be broadly interpreted as complementary health care practices.

The Complementary Care Center in Phoenix, Arizona, founded in 1993, has one of the most comprehensive programs of allopathic and alternative medicine. This center, according to program director Sam Benjamin, is one of a handful of clinics in the United States already practicing standard Western medical care combined with biofeedback, acupuncture, homeopathy, craniosacral therapy, guided visual imaging, and twelve other alternative therapies. Sometimes Benjamin prays with a patient or he writes healing words from the Bible and tapes them to a patient's pillow before surgery. Even the architecture of the center reflects this holistic approach with gently curved hallways and tear-shaped waiting areas.

Many people believe that alternative techniques, which are less invasive and therefore often take more time, may entail higher up-front preventive costs but in the long run will cost less by reducing tests, procedures, and hospitalizations. In 1997 Washington became the first state to require reimbursement by insurance companies for treatment performed by any licensed or certified health care practitioner of massage, acupuncture, and some thirty other techniques. For example, massage has shed its association with sex parlors and now is embraced as therapy with 17 percent of the adult U.S. population reported having massages in the past five years and 12 percent in the past twelve months.[27] Its use is growing exponentially.

The growth of alternative health care is phenomenal. Fifty-eight percent of HMOs planned to reimburse their members for alternative medical treatment by 1999.[28] Consider that the Oxford Health Plan serves 1.5 million people and has 550 practitioners of alternative medicine.[29] Half of the family practitioners in the country prescribe alternative medicine; $30 billion is spent on alternative therapies in the United States.

Thirty-four of 125 medical schools in the United States—including Harvard, Yale, and Johns Hopkins—now offer courses in alternative medicine.[30] Even the American Medical Association is urging its members to become better acquainted with alternative medicine. The World Congress on Complementary Therapies in Medicine represents an increasing mix of the Western medical establishment, Eastern practitioners, and herbal salespersons.

Folkloric Health Care Practices Rediscovered

Most people describe folkloric health care as traditional medicine. Medicine as we generally use the term is not appropriate. A more accurate term may be "folkloric health care practices," since they are related to a particular set of cultural practices and beliefs and do not employ modern health care techniques. They reflect "ways of protecting and restoring health that existed before the arrival of modern medicine";[31] from 65 to 80 percent of the world's population relies on traditional medicine. (It is now receiving recognition, as evidenced by the National Institutes of Health's Office of Alternative Medicine, which was designated by the World Health Organization as a Collaborating Center in Traditional Medicine.)

My personal experience with folkloric health care practices was rather negative while living for six years in the interior of Brazil in the 1960s. My second son, Nato, as a several-month-old baby, was steadily losing weight. Our neighbor said he had *mingua* (poverty, or dire lack of something; as illness, probably dietary deficiency or malnourishment) and unbeknownst to us took a drop of his blood to the local *curadeiro* to remove the bad spirit she thought was causing the condition.[32] Of course, from her perspective she was doing something helpful, following the practice of local custom. The widespread use of *curadeiros*, combined with poverty and lack of education, however, was one of the principal reasons for the low life expectancy. (I do not have figures for the remote area of Santa Catarina where we lived, but in the northeast of Brazil in the 1960s the average life expectancy was thirty-seven years.) Without medical advice our son could have died if we were left with the diagnosis of *mingua*. Instead we took a twelve-hour bus trip on dirt roads to Curitiba, Parana, where the doctor who examined him discovered he was allergic to cow's milk. We bought a goat, and after one week of goat's milk our son began to flourish. (We later switched to soy milk.) Of course, the neighbor was convinced that the *curadeiro* healed him.

One must acknowledge that some folkloric health care practices, for example, in Africa and China, can be quite effective. The black tea fungus, also known as "the Treasure," is used in Africa, Asia, and the former Soviet Union, making its way into the United States in places such as Wheeling, West Virginia. It is thought to be a cure-all for most everything. A former Peace Corps volunteer in Benin, West Africa, remembers drinking the tea in the village where she lived. The ripe fungus floats over the bucket of tea, growing bigger the longer it floats. Tea is poured directly from the bucket into cups for drinking. It has a pleasant, sweet-and-sour taste, and is slightly carbonated, like fermented apple juice.[33] The tea reportedly originated in the Caucasus region of the former Soviet Union where many of the villagers lived to be more than a hundred years of age, continued to do hard labor in the fields—and even reproduced children at that age! Nobody suffered from high blood pressure, heart disease, cancer, or tumors. All of the villagers drank the black fungus tea daily. A Japanese woman visiting the village took some of the fungus home with her. It spread in use in Japan before being introduced into China's Sichuan Province in 1945, and then Africa.[34]

REDISCOVERY OF LINK BETWEEN SPIRITUALITY AND GOOD HEALTH

An additional reason for the fullness of time for the expansion of the church's health ministry is the renewed interest in spirituality and health. The connection between these two was already noted in the resurgence of complementary health care practices whose more wholistic practices welcome the spiritual dimension. We have witnessed in the past few years a tremendous growth of interest in spirituality, spiritual development, spiritual disciplines, and spiritual formation, reflected by popular articles and new books, as well as seminary and medical school courses devoted to the subject. However, there is an important distinction between religious beliefs and practices, and general spirituality. "Spirituality" is a rather amorphous term with broad definitions. Some people who refer to spirituality are antireligious or antichurch, while others may attend the local Presbyterian or Roman Catholic church and be very comfortable with religious teachings and practices. It is instructive that as prestigious an organization as the World Health Organization added in 1998 the word "spiritual" to its definition of health.[35]

It is not surprising that this interest in spirituality has spilled over into the health field with a growing body of literature on spirituality and health. Dr. Larry Dossey, former cochairman of the panel of Mind/Body Interventions, Office of Internal Medicine, National Institutes of Health, wrote in his earlier book *Beyond Illness* about spirit and its connection with medicine: "Oddly, 'spirit' has seemingly thrived on being officially ignored in medicine in the scientific era, perkily asserting its presence in every doctor's encounter with a patient and in every patient's encounter with illness. For something so diaphanous, it has uncanny persistence."[36] Our habit of ignoring spiritual concerns in medicine has evolved not because physicians are more spiritually bankrupt than any other professional group, but for the quite simple reason that it seemed unnecessary to insert them in our scientific understanding of health and disease. Nowhere did they seem vital in unraveling the anatomical and physiological complexities of human beings, nor in prescribing proper therapies when the body went awry. "The tendency to ignore the spiritual domain reflected a basic economy of thought and doing which is part of the scientific ideal."[37] Dossey attempts in this book to trace the spirit's presence in medicine and connect it to the sense of service that doctors still have. His use of the word "spirituality" is more in the sense of human virtues or ideals.

In addition, there are those who translate an emotion like love as part of spirituality; writers such as Bernie Siegel refer to love, medicine, and miracles as in his book by that title.[38] Dossey, for example, believes that love forms a bond with the person who is prayed for, hence allowing us to heal at a distance. Unity, not separation, is fundamental. Yet love is no guarantee against sickness.[39]

Princeton Engineering Anomalies Research Center (PEAR), which has been studying anomalous human-machine interactions for nearly two decades, concludes that love is at the center of this interaction, this "blurring of identities between operator and machine" that influences output. The *scientific* message, PEAR observes, is parallel to the message of the patriarch of modern physics, Prince Louis de Broglie: "In loving ourselves, we can heal ourselves. In loving the world, we can heal the world."[40]

An increasing number of courses and workshops address the contribution of spirituality to healing. A symposium at Jacksonville, Florida, dealt with spirituality and pain. A Mayo Clinic conference in Rochester, Minnesota, for the paramedical and nursing communities specifically addressed scientific studies on the role of spirituality in care, noting that illnesses such as burnout are soul illnesses. The Mayo Clinic also has a number of didactic programs for the medical staff on how to break bad news to patients and their families. The clinic aligns this attempt to make medical care more humanistic with introducing spirituality into medicine, an interesting shift, given the fact historically that the spiritual is connected to the transcendent, not the human.

Edward Creagan, an oncologist at the Mayo Clinic, encounters no problems at all in dealing with spirituality, even when patients are avowed atheists. "Everybody has a spiritual dimension. We are not talking about *religion*, we are talking about *spirituality*," which means they avoid terms like "Christian care."[41] Chaplains are part of the total Mayo experience, fully salaried and part of the medical team; they handle some of the great questions of life and medicine as members of the hospital's ethics committee.

Therapeutic Touch Enters Mainstream Medicine

The three practices of therapeutic touch, psychic healing, and Silva mind control illustrate the interface of health and spirituality. One of the most popular practices of alternative health care that facilitates healing by accessing a person's energy field is therapeutic touch (TT).[42] A conservative estimate of fifteen thousand nurses use it in the United States,[43] and it is taught in more than seventy countries.[44] The technique of therapeutic touch was developed in the early 1970s by Dolores Krieger, a registered nurse and professor of nursing at New York University. She was the first person to study the laying on of hands in human subjects and, from it, developed a variation called therapeutic touch. Krieger hypothesized that hemoglobin would be a sensitive indicator of energy change and oxygen uptake, which serve as an appropriate test for the laying on of hands. In responding to critics of therapeutic touch she stated, "A study done ten years ago on post-operative patients found that wound healing was more rapid in patients who had TT."[45] Therapeutic touch is based on the assumption that human beings have complex patterns of energy and that disease is associated with a disorder or blockage of the energy flow both within the patient and between the patient and the environment. Author and nurse Karen Philigan explains that "body tissues are made up of molecules, which are composed of atoms, which are made of protons, neutrons and electrons, which produce energy. The electromagnetic field of a person is what is assessed during therapeutic touch."[46]

A *Life* cover story, "The Healing Revolution," opened with a description of a triple bypass operation at Columbia Presbyterian Medical Center in New York City. On one side is a cardiothoracic surgeon, and on the other is a nurse trained in therapeutic touch, directing the flow of energy to help the patient relax without touching him. Dr. Mehmet Oz, the surgeon, noted how inseparable were the patient's emotions and his health. Helen McCarthy, the nurse involved, was specifically trained in therapeutic touch. The sight of a surgeon and an energy healer working side by side in one of this country's most prestigious hospitals reflects an extraordinary détente in U.S. medicine.[47]

In order for therapeutic touch to be effective, "the healer must have a sincere intent to help another," says Philigan, who practices the technique. "He or she should also be in good health. When I have a cold, I cannot sense the field with my hands, and my energy flow is blocked." The patient also has a role to play by "deciding" how the energy he or she receives will be used rather than being a passive recipient of it. Under controlled laboratory conditions, distinct biological changes have been noted. The practitioner needs to be "centered" (a state of relaxation where all personal considerations are put aside). TT may not involve literal touching, but it is a way of experiencing or feeling the electromagnetic energy field of another person.[48] For this reason many discounted thirteen-year-old Emily Rosa's experiments, which challenged TT's effectiveness because her research did not take into account the needed bonding between patient and practitioner.[49]

Larry Dossey describes cases where therapeutic touch has been successful in healing wounds where standard treatments may not have been.[50] However, he expresses concern about an overreliance on alternative medicine, which may court disaster, while encouraging an attitude of acceptance of and gratitude to new methods that may allow miraculous cures to take place.[51] Although research has found that patients who follow an integrated program of allopathic and alternative medicine have less postoperative pain and anxiety, one must use both theological and scientific rigor in assessing the use of this and other innovative resources for healing.

Krieger's human studies were preceded in the early 1960s by Bernard Grad, a biochemist at McGill University. He collaborated with two other scientists in double-blind studies on mice and barley seeds. Grad wounded three hundred mice by cutting an oval of skin along the spine. He divided them into three groups. The first group was allowed to heal without outside intervention. Mice in the second group were individually held fifteen minutes, twice a day, by a well-known healer. Mice in the third group were held by medical students who did not profess to heal. After the sixteenth day, the wounded area of the second group treated by the healer was significantly smaller than the size of the wounds of the other groups. Similar results were found when barley seeds were soaked in saline solution to simulate a sick condition. Those watered with fluid from flasks held by the professed healer sprouted more quickly, grew taller, and contained more chlorophyll than the seeds in the control groups.[52]

Psychic Healing: Authentic or Quackery?

Healing as the transference of energy, more popularly known as psychic healing, is another newly studied form of healing at the juncture of spirituality and health. Mainline religious people are often uncomfortable with discussions about this topic. The question stems from whether the success of the psychic healer has more to do with the patient's faith in the process than in any objective or inherent power on the part of the healer.

I will have to confess my skepticism, having lived in Brazil up the road from a psychic surgeon named Arigo, "the surgeon of the rusty knife." Arigo, an uneducated Brazilian, performed surgeries without anesthetic using a kitchen knife. His "operations" were removing tumors, abscesses, and appendixes, and involved all manner of procedures. In addition, he used strange herbs and procedures, which he claimed were at the direction of a deceased German doctor who spoke to him in psychic revelations. John Fitzpatrick also was acquainted with Arigo in the 1970s and discusses the phenomenon of psychic healing rather sympathetically in his book *Create Your Own Health Patterns*.[53] Father Fitzpatrick worked in the same area of Brazil that I did. He concludes that Arigo and other spiritualists heal some people, fail to heal others, make other people worse, and temporarily heal others. While Fitzpatrick hedges his bets, William Nolen completely discredits psychic surgeons like Arigo as well as those from the Philippines.[54]

Odic Force Viewed Positively

Leslie Weatherhead, a famous London Methodist preacher in the mid-twentieth century, meanwhile deemed some psychic healing to be authentic and described one of its manifestations as radi-aesthetic energy or "odic force." The term "odic force" derives from Odin, the god of ancient Norse mythology whose power permeated everything in heaven and earth. Reichenbach, who was a chemist in Stuttgart from 1788 to 1869, first used this term. For him, "odic force" referred to emanations from a magnetized bar that "sensitives" described as a stream of light. It is detected in any substance undergoing change. The force has healing energy and accounts for the phenomenon of table-turning and passes made by the hands of the mesmerist.[55] Weatherhead believed this psychic energy accounted for the gifts of healing that some people possess. Healing is understood as a transfer of energy between the healer and the patient. The term "centering" is often used by healers to describe what they are doing by excluding all extraneous, distracting thoughts and feelings in order to assume an attitude of selflessness, a way of being instead of doing.[56] This begins to sound similar to therapeutic touch.

Mind over Matter

Another form of psychic healing is practiced by people who study Silva mind control. This method helps people learn to use their minds to control the outcome of events or healing (rooted in the popular phrase "mind over matter"). In 1975, Robert N. Miller, an industrial research scientist, and Philip B. Reinhard, head of the physics department at Agnes Scott College, ran experiments to determine if measurable energy was given off by the famous healer Olga Worrall. The researchers determined the energy could be measured at a distance of six hundred miles away.[57] These findings further corroborate Dossey's research.

The type of energy measured is a matter of some discussion. Olga Worrall referred to psychic energy as a "universal field" whose source is God; hence it is not Worrall but God who heals. The psychic can also see an aura that surrounds "the patient." The Russian Seymon Kirlian developed a technique to photograph the aura of animals and plants. We have heard of people talking to plants; perhaps this is not an eccentricity. Peter Knudtson and David Suzuki in their book *Genethics* discuss the Mayans' worshiping of corn, which in gratitude brought forth multicolored ears,[58] a graphic display of the so-called transfer of energy that Weatherhead noted between the healer and the patient.

Researchers at the PEAR Institute at Princeton University School of Engineering conclude that at present we have no theoretical model that explains the role of the conscious in the definition of physical reality and how psychic healing occurs. However, the fact that we do not understand how the conscious works is no basis to contest its effectiveness; there are many therapies that at first worked and later we understood why.[59]

SCIENTIFIC STUDIES OF RELIGIOUS BELIEFS AND PRACTICES

In addition to health care's incorporation of spirituality into its delivery systems are the growing number of scientific studies that provide information about the impact of religious beliefs and practices on health. We find ourselves navigating new territory, not being overconfident about the reliability of these studies yet recognizing the revolutionary potential of religious beliefs and practices as well as general spirituality on good health. These studies, despite our reservations, constitute the fifth reason this is the fullness of time for the church's health ministry. So consistent are studies' findings showing the beneficial effects of religious commitment on numerous and diverse health and health care outcomes that it may be prudent for physicians and appropriate for federal health policy makers to incorporate such perspectives in their treatment plans. Religion is a major factor in many people's lives. Despite protests that religion has been subsumed by secular society, "data from a thirty-five-year period of Gallup polls consistently indicates that 95 percent of Americans believe in God and 76 percent pray regularly."[60]

To many, the juxtaposition of scientific and religious practices is an oxymoron. However, modern science is beginning to consider the interpenetration of the physical and the nonphysical. The breakdown of a dualistic view of mind and spirit allows room for healing prayer that can often be grasped by the heart before it can be understood by the mind.[61] There is a deep reticence to submit God to the laboratory, to measure psychic energy in an ivory tower environment, or to sanction control studies about the power of prayer. It may seem sacrilegious or, at a minimum, not the topic for academicians and scientists.

We should not assume that God does not want to be studied as we analyze scientific studies showing the effect of religious beliefs and practices on healing. That view is rather presumptuous, as if we know what God wants. It may be important for us to study prayer scientifically to help us find answers to some of life's deepest questions.[62] We should not be afraid to submit the effects of prayer, laying on of hands, and other religious practices to scientific study just to protect the spiritual realm from deconstruction or a reductionist mode of thinking. Spiritual dimensions to healing ultimately may far exceed our ability to explain them even with our most sophisticated tools of inquiry.

I was first challenged to consider the juxtaposition of science and religious practices in 1983 by Dr. Elizabeth McSherry, a Harvard-trained pediatrician. She asserted that if the church was going to be involved in health ministries, it needed to translate its work into understandable language and methodology for the scientific and medical professions. The church should be able to measure outcomes in order to illustrate that the ecclesial body can be an effective center for healing.

McSherry has written many articles on this subject. Some of the early data she gathered[63] showed a reduction of 30 to 50 percent of hospital stays for Wholistic Health Centers, Inc., patients where the patient's spiritual dimension was cared for and managed.[64] The value of spiritual counseling was also demonstrated by a University of Virginia study of age and type of injury–matched orthopedic patients. The random assignment of a hospital chaplain for daily visits was the independent variable associated with a decrease in hospitalization days, amount of pain medication needed (to one-third the matched control group), and ward-based professional time.[65]

Additional studies have been cited, such as the Alameda study that covered 5,286 people since 1965.[66] The Graham study of white male heads of households in Evans County, Georgia, showed a consistent pattern of lower systolic and diastolic blood pressures, which was identified among frequent church attenders, independent of the effects of age, obesity, smoking, or social class.[67] Also cited have been a decrease in hypertension and an increase in longevity among Seventh Day Adventists and a branch of the Mormon Church.[68] More recent studies reinforce these earlier findings. Researchers at Johns Hopkins University have found cardiovascular disease significantly reduced by a lifetime of church attendance. Numerous other studies confirm that churchgoers live longer with lower rates of cirrhosis, emphysema, and arteriosclerosis. "Religious involvement greatly decreases drug use, delinquency, premarital sex and increases self-control for all age groups. In a 1985 study of girls, 9 to 17, less than 10 percent of those who attended religious services weekly reported drug or alcohol use, compared to 38 percent of the overall group."[69] "In a study of 87 depressed patients hospitalized for medical conditions like heart disease and stroke, those who scored high on a measure of 'intrinsic religiosity' recovered faster from depression than those who scored low on the scale."[70]

Moving from a few scattered studies of the effects of prayer and church attendance on physical health, two of the principal analysts of a more systematic collection of studies are Dale Matthews and Larry Dossey. In most instances, they are not conducting the research but reporting work done by credentialed scientists, which usually appears in peer-reviewed journals. The most comprehensive treatment is the four-volume work by Dale Matthews, David Larson, et al. at the National Institute for Healthcare Research (NIHR) on the faith factor in health and illness. Here their conclusions are reported but not verified by an independent review of the primary data, which is beyond the purview of this book.

The Faith Factor Analysis

Larson, formerly of the National Institute of Mental Health, is now president of the National Institute for Healthcare Research in Maryland. He is a psychiatrist and researcher who initiated the effort to collect and analyze hundreds of studies on the role of religion in physical, mental, emotional, and spiritual health. *The Faith Factor*, a collaborative effort by Matthews, Larson, and colleagues, summarizes the research of clinical abstracts, tracking religion and faith with different populations and illnesses; it is fascinating and thorough. In a nutshell, these studies tell us that faith and religion may be the most underrated medical factors and their effect can be measured scientifically.

The data-based studies for *The Faith Factor*'s four volumes of research used "acceptable clinical and religious variables with published methodologies in peer-reviewed journals."[71] Clinical abstracts were used to summarize and communicate relevant data. Patients' religious beliefs and practices were evaluated by applying scientific outcomes that are measurable and verifiable. *The Faith Factor* authors noted that "the level of religious commitment as measured by specific behavior such as church attendance and volunteerism needs to be assessed in addition to the measure of attitude and belief." They found that "the use of denominational preference as a measure of religiosity is not recommended because of the low explanatory power and utility of this measure." Some of these studies may have "overdrawn their case" because the samples used "highly religious students, parishioners and returning missionaries."[72] Longitudinal studies are needed in addition to control studies, which cover short periods of time.

Summary of The Faith Factor's Findings

The first volume includes 158 individual studies linking religious variables and clinical assessments of mental and physical health status. Volume 2 reviews 35 articles, mainly key field systematic reviews, which examine the various aspects of the relationship between religion and health (and mental health), with volume 3 providing 80 additional individual studies, and volume 4, another 100 research studies.

In 146 studies of the 158 abstracted in volume 1, 112 (77 percent) demonstrated that religion can positively influence health, 25 (17 percent) were neutral or mixed, and a minority, or 9 studies (6 percent), demonstrated negative effects from religious variables. "The positive effects of religious variables or commitment were found in every area including drug and alcohol use, psychological symptoms, physical symptoms and general health outcomes, and psychosocial variables including well-being measures."[73] The following is a summary of some of the findings that reflect the results of the summarized studies.

"The effect of religious commitment upon substance abuse included reduction of alcohol consumption in sixteen of the eighteen studies, nicotine in six of six studies (100 percent) and drug use in twelve of twelve studies (100 percent)."[74] This data is important, if not revolutionary, when you consider that in the United States annually 400,000 deaths are caused by tobacco and 100,000 deaths by alcohol.[75] Improved psychological health "included improvement in adjustment and coping in fourteen out of fifteen studies (93 percent)." Religious commitment "reduced the overall number of adverse psychological symptoms in eleven out of thirteen cases, including depression (twelve out of seventeen cases or 71 percent); hostility (four out of four cases); general anxiety (eight out of eleven cases); and death anxiety (ten out of fifteen cases or 67 percent)." In addition, "the effect of religious commitment on [extent or level of] physical symptoms and general health outcomes included improved general health (four out of five); reduced blood pressure (four out of five); improved quality of life in cancer (seven out of eight) and heart disease patients (four out of six); and increased survival (eight out of nine or 89 percent)." General well-being was positively correlated with religious variables such as "greater life satisfaction (92 percent), improved marital satisfaction (100 percent), and self-esteem (two out of four studies or 50 percent)."[76]

Reduction of Blood Pressure by Religious Practices and Spiritual Healing

The Faith Factor also examined studies that looked at a single health problem, such as high blood pressure. Between 1954 and 1984 there were twelve blood pressure studies reported by J. S. Levin and H. Y. Vanderpool in *Social Science and Medicine*. These studies included measures of religious commitment in "Benedictine and Trappist monks, Seventh Day Adventists, Mormons, and Zen Buddhist priests and others. Only one study compared Protestants, Catholics and Jews. The authors noted that in cross-religious affiliations, adherents of the more highly devout groups that restricted certain behaviors or diets had lower rates of hypertension."[77]

"Randomized, double-blind control trials of 'laying on of hands'" are another interesting area of study. In the *British Medical Journal* a study was reported in 1988 by J. J. Beutler et al. of patients with essential hypertension. In these studies the laying on of hands was "associated with greater patient well-being but no reduction in systolic or diastolic blood pressure compared with patients who were treated with healing at a distance. There was no correlation between increased well-being and reduction of blood pressure."[78]

Church Attendance and Good Health

One of the most extensive studies reported by *The Faith Factor* was conducted by G. W. Comstock and K. B. Partridge in 1972 to assess effects of church attendance on health and health behavior. The population survey was of 91,909 individuals in the general population of Washington County, Maryland. The conclusion of the study was that "frequency of church attendance is associated with significant reductions in morbidity and mortality from a variety of disease conditions."[79]

Another cross-sectional survey of patients registered at a health center in Glasgow, Scotland, studied the effects of church attendance on health. A random sample of the patient list was interviewed with 964 respondents aged sixteen or older. Adults with a religious allegiance to the Roman Catholic Church, the Church of Scotland, and other Protestant denominations had a 41 percent better physical, mental, and social outcome than their nonchurch counterparts.[80]

Religious Commitment and Drug Use in Adolescents

A 1984 study by C. K. Hadaway, K. W. Elison, and D. M. M. Petersen examined "the relationship between religious commitment and drug use and attitudes towards drug use among adolescents." The principal results of this study indicated that the student's "church attendance, parents' church attendance, personal importance of religion, personal prayer, orthodoxy, and obedience to parents are all inversely related to use of alcohol, marijuana, and other drugs and attitudes towards use of these substances. Respondents who believed religion to be extremely important were much less likely to drink at least once a week (8 percent versus 26 percent), use marijuana often (5 percent versus 23 percent), and use other illicit drugs (7 percent versus 25 percent) than those who believed religion to be 'not too important.'"[81]

A review of *The Faith Factor* raises the original questions: Can we measure God in the laboratory? Can faith be quantified? Do we shortchange spirituality if we reduce its effects to scientific studies? Our answers in part depend on how we understand the pursuit of knowledge. Are we cooperating with God or usurping God's domain? The entire subject of scientific studies of religion challenges the inexplicable nature of healing. This is central to our inquiry because it poses the question whether it is God's actions, which are inexplicable, or our lack of knowledge that impedes our understanding.

Larry Dossey's View on Religious Beliefs and Practices

These same questions are pursued by Larry Dossey and provide a slightly different perspective. Dossey's perspectives on the effects of prayer and spiritual healing are important since he has become such a popular figure in the field of holistic health. His main thesis is that we need to keep studying prayer scientifically because it is a powerful force even if we are not clear about its results. There are some indications that it is effective, but we need to improve the design of the protocols and broaden the populations being studied. Dossey is critical of the scientific rigor of a number of early studies. They claim positive correlations between prayer and improved health but cannot actually prove their claims. He seems to accept the premise that in time studies will legitimize prayer as part of medical treatments. He identifies himself not as religious or a member of a faith community but as someone interested in prayer because it works. Perhaps Dossey's most significant contribution is putting prayer and other religious practices on the health care agenda. His popularity causes people—who heretofore might have given slight consideration to such matters—to think about the power of prayer in healing.

Toward the end of his book *Healing Words*, Dossey states, "Although science has much to say about prayer, it raises more questions than it answers. The mysteries of prayer not only remain, they deepen."[82] Despite some positive results in scientific studies about prayer, what is essential is to affirm the importance and meaning of prayer in our lives. Prayer works in ways that are totally unmeasurable. However, that is not a reason to avoid studying it.

Dossey is particularly interested in understanding the role that prayer plays in a variety of illnesses. Yet his studies are not only of prayer but include an examination of psychic energy, imaging, meditation, and the phenomenon of nonlocal matter.

As part of Dossey's studies of prayer and its effects, he presents an analysis of the three eras of medicine: Era I from 1860 to about 1950 being body oriented; Era II from the 1950s, focusing on the mind-body connection; and Era III in the 1990s, the nonlocal, mind-body-spirit perspective we are currently experiencing, which defies explanations in ordinary, physical, reductionistic frameworks.[83]

Dossey's Era III view becomes the basis of the claim that through our thought processes we can "reshape" our "medical past." Prayer can be answered before it is even offered in the eternal now. The fact that good things happen to bad people and vice versa may be "time displaced" events.[84] This rather unusual view of time reminds us of Aquinas's teaching that for God, past, present, and future are all now. This is another way of challenging a linear view of time. In this context, Dossey believes that sometimes a medical test itself may become self-fulfilling, though he offers the intriguing possibility that if we pray fervently between the time of the test and our knowledge of its results, we may change the results to a positive outcome.

Are Prayer Experiments Ethical?

One of the underlying questions about these scientific studies is whether they are ethical. This issue needs to be explored from several perspectives. First, since prayer is a potent force, it can also be harmful. Knowing that a negative prayer is being directed toward a person, the "victim" can "live out" the harmful effects and actually die.[85] This could be considered parallel to the curses placed on people by witch doctors or voodoo initiates. Second, many of the experiments do not offer statistically reliable or significant data, so the question is, Are they justified?[86] What does it say about God who appears to favor one group over another? If "prayer works," we should see statistically more consistent results from studies. This brings us to the third ethical aspect concerning prayer: If it is proved efficacious and we fail to use it, are we being unethical? "So pervasive will its use become that not to recommend the use of prayer as an integral part of medical care will one day constitute medical malpractice."[87] Because Dossey is cochair of the NIH Alternative Medicine Center Panel on Mind/Body Interventions, his statement carries weight in the scientific community.

Conclusions Based on Dossey's Work

After having read Dossey's book and other studies, we stand on shaky ground if we try to argue that science has proved at this stage of the research the efficacy of prayer and religious beliefs as contributing to good health. The data are simply too mixed. As was mentioned previously, Dossey concludes that the early human studies conducted by pioneers such as R. B. Byrd were troubled by too many variables, and he suggests that the more recent, nonhuman studies by Daniel Benor, for example, show more promise because they reduce the possibility of positive results of nonlocal events (such as prayer and acts of consciousness) being due to chance.

Dossey asserts that science and spirituality can now operate side by side. Spiritual healing will be gradually accepted as Era III medicine is understood, which will lead to the use of prayer in the practice of scientific medicine. Continued research by credible scientists on the effects of prayer and other religious practices on good health is crucial. Then prayer may become one more tool in the armamentarium of medicine. Now doctors conclude prayer can do no harm, so why not let patients pray?[88]

As Christians, we can embrace Dossey's work but focus less on the person imaging and praying and more on the mysterious God who is the source of all healing. God uses prayer, medicine, surgery, faith, drugs, touch, or no means at all to show forth God's healing power. Dossey concludes that prayed-for patients may experience a sense of acceptance and peace. This may be the most important "result." Christ bids us to pray not because of the results, though certainly those are alluded to in Christ's promise that prayer can move mountains, but because in prayer we talk to God. How else can we open ourselves to God's presence and movement in our lives? Prayer is our way of connecting with the divine energy, which is the source of all healing. Healing comes not from the prayer but from the God to whom we pray.

We should not avoid studies of prayer and psychic healing. We should constantly push the frontiers of knowledge to their extreme. The quest for knowledge is a holy quest, and we need not be afraid where it will lead. It is in the application of that knowledge that we must uphold the moral guidelines for the good of the whole and the glory of God. However, Paul Ramsey was right that our moral measure may be in the things we refuse to do as well as the things we do.[89]

Yes, this is the fullness of time for the church's involvement in health care in new and exciting ways. However, the type of programs and services appropriate for religious communities is still being determined. Ascertaining which ones to embrace or eschew is the challenge to be considered in the next chapter.

3

Discerning and Defining Authentic Health and Healing Ministries

O nce the shift from the medical model of health care has begun, the challenge of what to accept and reject of the various forms and practices of healing remains. The question of discernment of health care practices and ministries is at several levels: (1) those within medicine are skeptical of complementary health care practices and of the church's role in health care; (2) those from conservative theological traditions are suspicious of energy healers and other complementary health care practices; (3) those within historical Protestant denominations are skeptical of faith healing; and (4) those in health ministries struggle over what to include or exclude under orthodox or authentic health and healing ministries. A discussion of authentic healing practices begins with understanding the working of God through nontraditional avenues of healing—or put another way, how we discern authentic healing practices.

As described in chapter 2, there is a new openness to the connection between faith and healing, spirituality and health. We welcome this movement, yet we need "to test the spirits." By taking the lead role in these matters, the church can help to shape health care in the twenty-first century rather than lag behind. New discoveries are being made daily about the marvelous interactions of body, mind, and spirit, which can result in "miraculous" healings. These events broaden our understanding of how God works in the world. Holistic and alternative health care practices are welcome when they bring improved health and well-being.

Where there is healing, there is God; God is the source of all healing. God is not limited to our understanding of how God works. God uses a variety of means to heal including faith as testified by Christ's healing miracles. The "faith" factor is an element in recovery, as was noted in the section on scientific studies in chapter 2. When someone believes in the healer such as the doctor, herbalist, mesmerist, psychic, or practitioner of therapeutic touch, the practices can have a healing effect because of the assistance from the patient's frame of mind.

We should not give the realm of healing over completely to medicine, to the doctors who in a sense have become the new priests. Their practices in some ways are as strange as the folk healers of whom we are so critical. They speak a strange language; use rituals of inspection of feces and urine, blood-letting, and diet; and prescribe nasty-tasting medicines. Both scientific medicine and alternative health care practices direct themselves toward the sick individuals rather than the social circumstances that make them sick. Of course, quacks and charlatans may also prey on the desperately ill, many of whom will follow any untested treatment offering a ray of hope. Reliance on theological and medical experts who can assist us in the discernment process is crucial, while remembering "skepticism is the chastity of the mind."[1]

CRITICISMS OF COMPLEMENTARY HEALTH CARE PRACTICES REMAIN

Not everyone accepts complementary health care practices, and skeptics abound both from medicine and from theology. The National Council against Health Fraud describes alternative medicine as complete nonsense and asserts there is no proof of its effectiveness. *The Reader's Guide to Alternative Health Methods,* coedited by Steven Barrett, uses the word "quack" 209 times in its first thirty-six pages.[2] Critics of alternative health care argue that most of its research is methodologically flawed, since it does not consist of the double-blind, placebo-controlled studies that are medicine's gold standard. Practitioners of alternative health care may miss a severe illness that only conventional medicine can effectively address. Allopathic medicine asserts that its regime of drugs and surgeries works independently of the patient's beliefs about them. There is a confidence born of repeated successes, which alternative practitioners cannot claim. For example, many medical practitioners believe Andrew Weil's methods would never pass an Institutional Review Board, though they concede that much of his advice—including exercise, eating healthy foods, and relax-ation—is sound. However, practitioners of alternative health care claim that critical doctors are threatened by an integrative approach to medicine because it takes away some of their control and empowers the patient.

Criticisms also come from the religious side. Some Christians are con-cerned that these practices are rooted in Eastern religions or New Age spirituality. Others believe they may even be connected with demons.[3] In many ways, the embracing of these practices reflects the bankruptcy of Western Christianity's healing ministries. Parish nurses, for example, are divided over their use with some of them belonging to the Holistic Nursing Association, which embraces these practices, while others distance themselves completely from the movement. Among clergy the reaction is mixed. Some clergy receive training, for example, in energy healing and practice in their churches or in a private practice. A number of seminarians use complementary health care as part of their personal health practices.

A RENEWED INTEREST IN THE ROLE OF FAITH IN HEALING

Some people would include prayer and faith as a type of spiritually based complementary health care practice. The interest in spirituality and health has caused doctors to take a closer look at the link between faith and healing. The most common link between spirituality and health concerns "faith healing"; by this we mean the contribution of a person's faith to improved health whether of a mental, physical, or emotional nature. The irony today is that while many Protestant churches and pastors are skeptical of faith healing, the medical profession is viewing it with new respect. According to a 1996 survey of the American Academy of Family Physicians, 99 percent of doctors believe there is an important relationship between the spirit and the flesh.[4] "I think this is a historic time," said Dr. Dale Matthews, a professor at Georgetown Medical School. "The spiritual traditions of healing will be joined with surgery and pharmaceuticals. I think we're entering the era of prayer and Prozac."[5] New diagnostic techniques enable medicine to address spiritual health problems. Health care professionals are paying new attention to the spirituality and health link.[6]

The Spiritual-Disorder Diagnostics Taxonomy for nurses, for example, includes questions about a patient's view of God, feelings of religious-based guilt, and so forth. The use of spiritual assessment instruments in clinical settings is growing. Many addiction treatment programs highlight spiritual as well as physiological causes. Centers like the Psychiatric Institute of Washington conduct courses on spiritual concerns and mental health. Edward Creagan observed, "Now we have to be both high-tech and high-touch."[7]

As previously mentioned, several mainstream magazines, including *Time* and *Life* in 1996 and 1997, carried lead stories on this newly appreciated phenomenon of spirituality, faith, and health with pictures of healing angels and heaven.[8] These stories reported the past neglect of religious and spiritual factors in U.S. health care. We can no longer ignore the mind-body-spirit connection, for it is not only real but measurable. Perhaps for this reason the psychiatric community is now paying more attention to religion and spirituality. According to Dr. Francis Lu of the University of California at San Francisco, many psychiatrists once either ignored religion or considered it a form of psychopathology. Now they are recognizing the importance of spirituality.[9] Study after study shows that spirituality increases longevity while decreasing destructive life patterns. Those without any strength or comfort from religion had almost three times the risk of death compared to those with at least some strength and comfort.[10]

Not only faith in religion but faith in the healer has always been an important ingredient in the healer's effectiveness. For example, Western physicians working with the Ibo tribe in Nigeria had limited success in healing villagers because of their suspicion of the physicians' practices. However, doctors from the Ibo tribe who were trained in Western medicine and combined it with native juju healing rituals were much more effective.[11] This view is parallel to Dossey's perspective that the doctor's faith in his practices and the patient's faith in the doctor have equal power to heal. In other words, faith may be the source of effectiveness of treatment on the part of either the doctor or the patient.

John Fitzpatrick similarly assessed the results of healers such as Kathryn Kuhlman. He believes that people may not stay healed because of a relapse of their belief in their healing, or their need for their illness, which perhaps blocked inner healing and peace.[12] He points out that faith and hope are linked and that faith generates hope and hope expectancy, which can bring profound emotional and psychological changes. Sister Justa Smith, a biochemist and enzymologist, carried out control studies of healing by a psychic named Mr. E whose power was directed toward wounded mice and plants.

> During the initial experiment—which lasted three weeks under scientifically controlled conditions—Mr. E consistently increased the activity of depressed enzymes, to a statistically significant degree, by the laying on of hands. The enzymes not treated by him did not regain activity. The same experiments done by people who did not claim to have healing power made no change in the enzymes. Smith concluded that there must have been a transference of energy but could not determine what kind of energy it was.[13]

Without reviewing the protocols and scientific rigor firsthand, however, Fitzpatrick's conclusions may be premature.[14]

Protestant Churches Skeptical of Faith Healing

While the Church of England is more systematic and ecclesial in its attempt to discern orthodox healing ministries, Americans in the historic Protestant denominations seem to be clearer what it is not, that is, television evangelists' healing services, slaying in the spirit, accounts of miraculous healing, or even the conducting of "healing" services. The discomfort of most Protestants with faith healing spills over into their whole assessment of what is authentic, orthodox, or even acceptable in a health ministry.

As we wrestle with the subject of discernment about authentic healing practices, at the center of this question is the assessment of faith healing. Popular writers and physicians have a renewed interest in faith healing. (See, for example, the Larson et al. *Faith Factor* studies.) Traditionally, we have linked spirituality and health by referring to "faith healing." However, this term has become virtually synonymous with what is practiced by the television evangelists and charismatic healers.

Faith healing usually refers to the contribution of a person's faith to improved health whether of a mental, physical, or emotional nature. The danger with faith healing is that it may shift the emphasis from connecting ourselves to God, who is the source of all healing, to concentrating on self. Our response should be shown in perseverance and in patience as we slowly overcome our disabilities. Fear, the opposite of faith in God, bogs us down in the present so we cannot move forward.[15]

Unfortunately, most people reduce religion's contribution to healing to an individual's faith or the community's prayers. Faith healing seems to refer to some esoteric activity that happens outside of time or space, to random events that occur to pilgrims on the way to Lourdes, or to a person with cancer healed at an emotional service. This random approach only raises questions about a God who is supposed to be equally concerned about all creation.[16]

Since we are living in a technological, scientific age, we need to approach faith healing in a different way. In New Testament times the spoken word had a great deal more power than it has today. If Jesus said, "Be healed," people believed it would happen. For cultures before the invention of the printing press, oral tradition was central to people's sense of self; hence words were more treasured. Today we seek verification and rational methods and explanations for the phenomenon of healing. Faith's triumphs are wrought through suffering and sacrifice. We must acknowledge that until some of the religious superstitions were put aside, many of the scientific insights that led to certain cures were not possible. For example, the early medical pioneers who tried vaccines on themselves before using them on patients may fulfill more fully what we mean by Christian healers than the faith healers who carry out a ministry with little cost to themselves.[17]

Scripture Affirms the Role of Faith in Healing

Even though there are misunderstandings about faith healing, distinguishing between glory-seeking faith healers and Jesus' use of people's faith in his healing miracles is important. The Scripture testifies that God may use a person's faith and prayer as vehicles for healing. "Daughter, your faith has made you well [whole]" (Luke 8:48). The faith of others may also be important. (See, for example, the story of the paralyzed man whose friends' faith was crucial to his healing, Matt. 9:1–8.) As we pray, humble faith is essential, especially as we struggle to understand the nature of the person's problem so prayer may be specific. Faith may open up a person to God's healing power, but it is God, not faith, who heals. The popularized faith healing approach may distort, as well as stop short of, a full understanding of the health ministry of the church.

Although there are forty healing miracles by Jesus cited in the Christian Scriptures, two-thirds of the Gospel healing stories lack any mention of faith. These include the man in the synagogue (Mark 1:23–26), the man beside the pool (John 5:2–9), and the man who was blind from birth (John 9).[18] Faith, as reliance upon God, is extremely important in healing prayer, but to insist on a strict connection between faith and healing is not reflected in the accounts of healing in the Christian Scriptures.[19]

Problems with the Faith Healing Approach

There are several problems with the popularized faith healing approach to illness, which is often isolated from a sound theology and a broad health ministry. Faith healing most often refers to healing at public services held outside the general worship life of the church. The first problem with faith healing is that it distorts the concept of the body. A dualistic or monistic outlook often lurks behind faith healing. Dualists among faith healers resemble the Gnostics of the second century who declared matter and the body to be evil (or demon possessed). Salvation and healing depend upon escaping from the body, the prison house of the flesh, and attaining repose wholly in spiritual matters. In this approach physical healing, for example, of cancer, would not be sought, but spiritual healing through the turning of the cancer's pain and suffering into suffering for Christ's sake.

Alternatively, Christian Science healers are monists who believe that matter and the body are not real. Sickness is an illusion, and healing is a question of attaining the right frame of mind. Either way, faith fails to honor and reckon with the body as a gift of God and to interpret sickness in the context of the whole person, an ensouled body. (A point worth noting is that Christian Scientists have reminded us of the importance of belief in God's power to heal, which was lost in many denominations.)

A second problem is that faith healing personalizes healing so that the patient or the faith healer, not God, is considered the source of healing.[20] When faith healing refers to the patient as producing a desired effect by the right kind of faith, it is misleading and for this reason should not generally be promoted. We need to connect with God, who is the source of all healing.

Third, faith healing may foreclose medical care. Its dualistic perspective suggests that the person who is spiritual enough, prays hard enough, and has enough faith needs no doctors. This view can lead to serious consequences, including the denial of symptoms and the refusal to receive treatment or even examination. A patient may avoid using the medical care that could in fact provide healing. This is especially true of those in acute psychological distress who may claim a temporary cure of an imaginary illness and never address the underlying causes of their illness.

Faith healers may misrepresent the Christian gospel with a bastardization of Christ's healing ministry. They take one instrument that Christ used—that is, faith—and claim it is the cause of healing. Christ's ministry was diverse and varied. Instead of eliminating medical care and health professionals, we need to integrate them with the church's resources. Jesus may have had more in common with physicians than with modern faith healers. Jesus did not advertise that he was about to hold a healing service, but quietly healed out of compassion, without advance publicity.

Fourth, faith healing creates false expectations; it trivializes hope; it promises, cruelly, that with enough faith anyone can be cured. Faith healers use the same method in every case, and they blame failure on the patient's lack of faith. If a patient is not cured, his depression is increased. He may deduce that religion is no good, the pastor is a liar, his own faith is weak, or God plays favorites. The patient who remains sick becomes a two-time loser—she still has the disease, and others suspect that her faith is inadequate. The guilt and despair may be worse than the original disease.[21]

Fifth, faith healing disconnects healing from the total life of the church when it separates healing services from general worship. Properly understood, the regular Sunday worship service is a healing service. This view prevails in many churches in England where healing is seen as part of the total sacramental life of the Anglican Church. This broader perspective avoids the dangers that may accompany public healing services if they are not within the context of the parish life with a known pastor and a community of believers.[22] Weatherhead warns about the emotionalism of the faith healing service with its sense of expectancy and excitement of the crowd. Based on a hysterical type of patient, the symptom, not the cause, can disappear. Often, these cures are temporary. But even worse, according to Weatherhead, is that one symptom may be permanently removed, and another, more severe one may follow.[23]

Finally, faith healing encourages an errand-boy image of God. God becomes an instrument of our needs rather than the source and ground of our being. In the Garden of Gethsemane Jesus asked for his heart's desire, but he was also ready to give over his own desires to God's will. This is the difference between submission and surrender—giving up and giving over.[24] Our prayer for healing should always be within the context of God's will and purpose in our lives.

Morris Maddocks has a more positive view of public healing services when they are within the context of a worshiping community. These healing services incorporate communion and the laying on of hands. As the Eucharist is celebrated within the context of a community, so should anointing and the laying on of hands. The Eucharist, however, should be the climax of the service. These practices then ground the healing services in the historic worship life of the church.[25]

AUTHENTIC HEALTH MINISTRY

The second aspect of discernment regarding which health ministries are orthodox is even more problematic. How do we discern true and false health ministries? Who is in a position to make such a judgment? What criteria do we use? Are our judgments based on a certain religious orthodoxy? How do we search for new directions? What is orthodox in one decade may become heresy in the next or vice versa.

Some guidelines are available to us. When Jesus, for example, was asked, "Are you the Messiah?" he cited results as the evidence of his claims: "The blind receive their sight, the lame walk, the lepers are cleansed, the deaf hear, the dead are raised, and the poor have good news brought to them" (Matt. 11:5). If this is the fullness of time for the church to recover its health ministries, what do we mean by "health ministries," and how do we assess what is authentic or legitimate? Health ministries generally involve organizations, programs, or initiatives. Healing ministries imply sacramental or liturgically oriented ministry. Discernment of the church's role in a health and healing ministry involves two questions: What is authentic, and what is orthodox?

The first question from the Christian perspective concerns which of the holistic, alternative, folkloric, and scientific health care practices are authentic, which ones can be embraced. "Authentic" is defined as what brings about positive healing; what is true and effective; what works, not what measures up to a certain objective standard.

The second question concerns the orthodoxy of healing movements and health ministries themselves; that is, what is true or false. "Orthodox" refers to right practices, which are historically and biblically grounded in the Christian church's teaching and practice.

The challenges of discernment in both arenas are extremely difficult. Authenticity rather than orthodoxy is our focus; the latter often has become the basis for witch-hunts, schisms, divisions, judgmental attitudes, and a host of unhealthy practices. Fundamentalists, in the name of orthodoxy, may banish other Christians from the church, saying they are not true believers because, for example, they do not hold to the inerrancy of Scripture. Liberals may practice their own brand of orthodoxy, claiming that if *all* practices are not accepted, one cannot be a real Christian.

Anglican Church Struggles over Authenticity

The Church of England in several of its Lambeth Conferences has wrestled with how to discern authentic health ministries. The Archbishops' Commission report in 1958 examined the various terms for healing ministry: "spiritual healing," "faith healing," and "divine healing." It settled on "the Church's ministry of healing" to emphasize the church's interest in the healing of the whole person. Terms such as "faith healing" imply that only certain methods of healing are spiritual or that only those with special gifts of healing within the church can heal or that a faith healer has special power—all these terms contain dangers. Hence the Church of England positioned itself in the center of the conversations about healing without an outright rejection of charismatic and deliverance ministries.[26]

Many Church of England members have been quite responsive to charismatic healers like John Wimber, in large part owing to Anglican priest David Watson, a renowned British evangelist, who worked extensively with Wimber. (Watson died several years ago of cancer.) More recently, the Churches' Council for Health and Healing had to decide, as various groups applied for membership, whether the ministries of deliverance and more charismatically organized groups should be accepted; they included them.

The recent revival of the healing ministry within the Church of England is not a cause for rejoicing for all people; some people within the church are skeptical about this revival.[27] Furthermore, there are so many different kinds of ministries that it is difficult to address them as a single unit. As previously mentioned, two of the dominant types of healing ministries in the United Kingdom are the sacramental and the charismatic. The first was represented by the Guild of Health founded in 1904 by Anglo-Catholics within the Church of England. This tradition is well represented by such people as Morris Maddocks and Christopher Hamel Cooke with their emphasis on the sacraments. The Institute of Religion and Medicine was founded to counterbalance the faith healing movement, largely imported from the United States. It was clearly aligned with the mainstream of the Church of England and the Royal Society of Medicine; the church's role was seen as following a sacramental ministry. Of course, not only the sacraments but also worship, prayer, and spiritual formation are included in this type.

The charismatic healing ministry has its roots in the nineteenth-century revivalism in the United States. For the Pentecostal, healing miracles occur through the power of the Holy Spirit. According to Stephen Pattison, this healing movement has been greeted with skepticism by the "mainline" churches, but Pentecostalism is the fastest-growing religious movement worldwide. The concern of the Church of England and others is that the charismatic healing ministries were in some instances connected to big business and right-wing politics in a movement called power evangelism and power healing: "The charismatic movement and religious healing are not throwbacks to some better time like the apostolic age. They are phenomena of our own age."[28] For some church leaders the charismatic approach creates a dichotomy between the social and the personal dimensions of the gospel so that justice issues of health care for all are totally neglected. These health ministries seem to be stuck in a time warp of attempting to re-create the healing ministry of apostolic times rather than relating it to the current scene.

The Church of Scotland addressed the question of authentic healing ministries by asking each presbytery to set up an informal review panel. These panels consist of members of the medical profession and clergy who review requests by groups for recognition. The criteria stipulate: "The ministry takes place in the name of the church and from within it as one of the healing ministries it can offer; the person ministering goes 'in the name of the Church' and is affirmed because of that; the person to whom ministry is given has some sense of confidence that the ministry has been given authority."[29]

This approach to discernment begins with defining what qualifies as health ministries. The Holy Spirit is the source of all gifts and especially the gifts of healing. Healing ministry includes prayer and intercession, blessing by the laying on of hands, anointing, healing of relationships, healing of memories, counseling, and spiritual direction (complementary medicine in Duncan's vocabulary). These gifts of healing are given for our growth in grace and nearness to God.[30]

C. Gordon Scorer, another British theologian, has addressed this issue by suggesting five tests of authentic Christian healing: (1) there is no symbol that is unnecessarily odd, for example, a revered object such as the bone of a saint since this is not part of the accounts of miraculous healing in the Christian Scriptures; (2) the believing Christian offers a fervent prayer; (3) the person doing the healing does not call attention to herself but stays in the background, unlike the showmanship style of many television evangelist–type healers; (4) a special commission is given by God to the healer such as Peter received at the Temple gate (Acts 3:1–11) and Paul at Lystra (Acts 14:8–11); and (5) healing miracles are followed by the presence of awe, fear, and the worship of God as was true in the Christian Scriptures.[31]

Duncan offers a slightly different approach to the discernment by describing the marks of authentic health ministry: the healing ministry must be (1) encompassed in prayer; (2) built, founded, and grounded in the Word of God; and (3) constantly guided by the Holy Spirit.[32]

DISCERNMENT REQUIRES DEFINING HEALTH MINISTRY

While offering a critique of the more sensational types of faith healing scenarios is important and giving general guidelines for authentic healing ministry is helpful, even more crucial is defining what constitutes authentic healing ministry. This task involves defining health ministry and discussing the health-related needs and areas the church is uniquely equipped to address. Health ministry involves churches as either sponsors or partners where faith, religious practices, and spiritual concerns are considered part of health care. It meets broad health-related needs and is founded, supported, or related to a church or religious group or body.[33]

The Health Ministries Association defines health ministry in a faith community as a wholistic approach to health that builds on the strengths of both the congregation and the community; it emphasizes wellness, health promotion, and disease prevention; encompasses congregational and community resources and partnerships; and focuses on body, mind, and spirit for the health and healing of the community. More broadly, health ministry involves empowerment, helping individuals, families, and communities help themselves and others through education, prevention, and advocacy. Health ministry is a church-based cooperative effort of individuals, hospitals, and other health agencies interested in an integrated understanding of health.[34]

Style of Church Health Ministry

Defining what we mean by health ministry has as much to do with its style as with the concrete programs and projects offered. In sharp contrast to marketplace medicine, the church's contribution to health care should be marked by concern for the person in need regardless of race, sex, age, or socioeconomic status. Christ identified himself with the sick: "I was sick and you took care of me" (Matt. 25:36; Luke 10:29–37). The parable of the good Samaritan provides a paradigm for this type of health care. Compassion was the motivating force for all the subsequent acts of this health minister par excellence as he ministered to the total needs of the person. What did the good Samaritan do? First, he showed compassion to the man who had been beaten by robbers and left half dead by the road-side. Because of his compassion, he

> treated the man's physical injuries;
> found him a bed;
> provided him with food;
> stayed with him during the initial crisis;
> paid the man's bills; and
> made provisions for his ongoing care.

In the same way that the good Samaritan reached out to care for his neighbor, the health and healing ministry of the church should glorify God through meeting people's needs on many levels. There are three interrelated levels to ministry to the sick: charitable, charismatic, and sacramental.[35] The ministry of healing and the promotion of health ulti-mately depend on reaching out in compassion to suffering people.

EFFECTIVE AREAS FOR THE CHURCH'S HEALTH MINISTRY

Advocating the role of the church as a health institution does not mean that the church should meet all health-related needs. It can respond effec-tively to health needs that touch the most sensitive parts of people's lives; meeting them constitutes a fundamental part of a congregation's ministry.

Meeting these health needs applies both to church members and to those on the periphery of the church's ministry. This ministry creates an opportunity for outreach and service beyond the membership of the church. Some persons may have no contact with a support community or caring fellowship. They may have found the church irrelevant or boring. They may desire counseling and education but are unsure and anxious about how to proceed. They may not understand the church's role in health and healing. The following are some suggested areas of health ministries in which the church can function effectively.

Creation of a Loving, Supporting Community

Concern, support, and the presence of others are very important in the healing process. A person in isolation can languish in loneliness and guilt. The church provides a resource for liberating people from "exaggerated individualism" and the isolation of contemporary life. The church functions as a community of acceptance and reconciliation. It can testify to the love and healing of God, which are available at all times, not just in moments of crisis. The power of forgiveness, communication, and companionship can often prevent, arrest, and alleviate disease. As was noted earlier, health is not simply an individual achievement but a harmony with the wider community. The *shalom* of the Hebrew Scriptures was not only inner peace and harmony, but wholeness in relation to one's world.

The church as an institution, which is multigenerational and intersects a person's life at various points, has an opportunity for assistance. Traditional functions of counseling, Bible study, religious education, prayer, and worship have tremendous healing potential. The church can celebrate the marvel of good health at all seasons of a person's life.

Healing communities are communities of people who know they need healing; they are communities of healers, and they are communities in the process of being healed. Churches are called to be obedient to the Spirit's healing activity in their midst where the Spirit is called down as a healing, reconciling force.[36] "Without the local fellowship, the ministry of healing is like a specialist medical service which has no hospitals and no public health clinics."[37]

The church can be both a caring community and an extended family to the patient. The communication of concern and interest can mitigate loneliness. The contribution of real assistance by cooking, baby-sitting, shopping, and helping with job placement can increase comfort to the patient. Comfort conveyed to the dependents of the patient for whom she usually cares can reduce her feelings of anxiety and guilt. In addition to concrete acts, visitation of the homebound sick and persons with disabilities extends the church's loving community as a place of healing. Visitation and counseling of the sick, however, may require special training of church members because deep emotions often surface in caring for the sick, in both the patient and the church members, risking a negative impact if poorly handled.

Spiritual Insights about Sickness and Health

The relationships between sin and sickness, faith and science, medicine and religion, pastor and physician, nurse and other health care professionals, surface when one is ill. When death and illness strike, people ask, "Where is God? Why is God silent when the righteous suffer? How can I endure in the midst of pain? How can I go on living as an altered person, either from injury or from catastrophic illness? How can I survive in the midst of pain? How can I tolerate a life with permanent disabilities or with the knowledge of a terminal illness?" My companion book *Redeeming Marketplace Medicine: A Theology of Health Care* discusses these questions in more depth, but suffice it to say, one turns to the church to understand the underlying meaning of health and sickness. Religion is assumed to answer these problems that medicine avoids.

Motivation to Change Lifestyle Patterns

Stress, burnout, hypertension, addiction, depression, and other health-defeating behaviors plague many individuals. People are concerned about the management of the total lifestyle, general health, and spiritual growth and development. Problems may arise in a variety of areas including stress reactions (such as headaches, backaches, ulcers, insomnia, hypertension), nutrition, use of addictive substances, interpersonal relationships, human sexuality, work, and personal and professional goals.

The church historically has been a strong force in urging health-enhancing lifestyles. The Methodist prohibitions against smoking and drinking had a substantial impact on the habits of eighteenth-century workers—to the point that Professor Robert Morrison of Cornell University and MIT looked back nostalgically to John Wesley as one of the "greatest public health officers" whom we could well use again today.[38] We need to be motivated to replace health-defeating with health-enhancing lifestyles.

Celebration of Health in All Stages of Life

Health is not merely the absence of disease, nor does healing consist only of curing. Healing includes a wide variety of activities that move us toward wholeness. There are ways of improving our health through prevention and a wellness orientation, which the Christian faith can provide at any point of the age span. The church, where we experience all seasons of our lives from baptisms to marriages to funerals, is the ideal institution to celebrate the stages of life. Our definition of health may change as we age.

The church has a special responsibility for the last season of life, for the elderly in our society, who are often marginalized and neglected. It can emphasize their contributions and worth, while society applauds only the young and the trim.

Provision of Integrated Health Care

From the Judeo-Christian perspective, health care should be wholistic and integrated; a person's spiritual, physical, emotional, and mental health needs should be included in any health care plan. Direct health services can be provided by the church based on whole person health care. The church can influence medical and theological education to equip professionals to use these new approaches. Teams of pastors, physicians, nurses, and other health-related professionals need to be developed using models like Westberg's Wholistic Health Centers. If wholistic health care is to happen, trained personnel are needed.

In addition, the laity should be equipped for health ministry. Deacons and other church officers can be trained to visit the hospitalized and homebound persons, provide some support services and referrals for the ill, counsel the bereaved, and assist in crisis intervention. Men and women already recognized as leaders in the church may enhance their skills to work with health care professionals and community agencies to meet health-related needs. They can be trained by programs such as the Stephen Ministries.[39] As chronic conditions increase, producing a need for home health care, church volunteers can provide an important supplement to medical personnel services.

We must not forget the support of traditional health care professionals and limit our support only to groundbreaking programs. Health care professionals' calling is both spiritual and medical. Their needs include affirmation of their professional work; support in dealing with the consequences of medical decisions when disease or death may claim a patient; setting of personal and professional priorities; and resolution of conflicts between personal and professional codes. Ethically and spiritually mature health care practitioners may do the most to strengthen the church's health ministry. Historically, the reassuring presence of nurses at times of illness existed long before the parish nurse program or other health ministries.[40]

Decision Making Concerning Health Care Options

One of the key issues is how to achieve quality health care at a reasonable cost. We face choices about health care, not only ways to reduce health care costs, but the choices of a physician and the type of health care plan. Navigating the health care swamp is not easy. Church-based health maintenance organizations that match patients and doctors by values and beliefs instead of geography or class could lower costs and improve doctor-patient relationships. As we noted earlier, people who follow religious practices have far superior health indices and access the health care system much less frequently. In addition, we need assistance in assessing our rights and responsibilities once in the patient-physician relationship.

Resolution of Bioethical Quandaries

Quandary issues are the seemingly insoluble choices between the right or good decision in a difficult situation. Technological medicine has developed at such a rapid rate, our ethics have been left far behind. Some of the bioethical quandaries we face include teenage pregnancy, abortion, technologically assisted parenthood (including surrogate motherhood), genetic counseling, organ transplants, gene therapies, and life-extending technologies. Questions arise concerning removal of a comatose teenager or cancer-ridden octogenarian from life supports; physician-assisted suicide for persons who are terminally ill; treatment for an alcoholic aunt or a nephew on drugs; and other decisions that affect the health and lives of friends and family. A theological framework and ethical principles can be provided through education and counseling by local church pastors and leaders to assist us in making reasoned choices.

Support, Compassion, Advocacy, and Assistance for Marginalized Persons

Certain illnesses and diseases are often labeled as unacceptable or beyond our area of concern. In this latter category those with AIDS, drug addiction, mental illness, or certain types of disabilities often are shunned by society. These people marginalized by virtue of their illness or medical condition may not receive the top medical treatment or, in fact, any health care; the tragic reality is that the church often ostracizes them. The church can become the voice for such powerless people and provide concrete assistance.

Fair Allocation of Health Care Resources

Assuring a decent fair minimum of health care resources for all persons, especially for the underserved and poor, is a crucial need in our society where there are millions of medically uninsured persons. In a climate of managed care, only the employed and rarely sick can expect adequate health care. Public policy initiatives, institutional restructuring, and personal sacrifice are needed to solve the current problems. The church that represents all strata of society is uniquely equipped for this mission. It needs to speak forth and implement equitable distribution of health care.

Advocacy of Health Care Reform

The health needs of people are not met by simply delivering medical resources. The underlying structures of society that prevent all people from receiving a decent fair minimum of care must be changed. We need to speak forth as the prophets of old against exploitation, injustice, and prejudice, and stand with those in need. However, we must first earn the right to protest and change society by gaining the trust and confidence of others by our acts of kindness and mercy. Concrete programs that meet real needs are necessary. Pronouncements from the pulpit and position papers from the church hierarchy will not make our voices heard. Work from the grassroots level and advocacy for real health care reform on every level are necessary.

Use of the Church Building

Although the ministry of the church by its members is preeminent in understanding the church as a healing community, the use of the church building cannot be overlooked. Many church buildings are underutilized, but eminently well suited to establishing and conveying a healing ministry. They are familiar places in the community; people are accustomed to going there for worship and other assistance. A person's rites of passage often take place there—baptism, confirmation, marriage, funeral. The building's use for a joint theological/medical ministry of healing fits and completes the church's mission as a healing community. Providing space for addiction recovery programs, day care centers, Meals-on-Wheels, respite care centers, and even health clinics carries forward the church's health ministry.

CATEGORIES OF HEALTH MINISTRIES PROGRAMS

By understanding the healing ministry of the church in these broader arenas, Christians and other people of faith can be encouraged to begin an active and effective health ministry. Part of analyzing the effective areas for a church-based health ministry is the determination of its range of activities, programs, and categories. As a way of analyzing the church's role, four categories of health ministry are recommended: sacramental/liturgical/devotional; educational; support/advocacy; and direct health services. These collectively may be understood to represent complementary health care practices. A local congregation, or group of churches, in collaborative partnership with the community may explore the possibility of implementing programs in some or all of these areas to assure balance in their health ministry. Resource organizations can assist the church to implement its health ministry.

Liturgical/Sacramental/Devotional

Liturgical ministries include the development and dissemination of resources for services of healing and anointing, the administration of sacraments, the practice of prayer, the ministry of deliverance, the holding of retreats, the proclamation of the Word, and the general worship life of the local congregation. These ministries also provide resources for recognition of the various passages of life that focus on restoring wholeness and well-being for an individual or community of faith.

Educational

The educational ministry is based on an integrated philosophy of health that addresses the underlying questions of health and sickness; the information and motivation about how to enhance health-affirming patterns of life including lifestyle changes; decision making about general health care options; the resolution of quandary issues; and the training for integrated health care.

An educational ministry develops, organizes, and administers programs or materials designed to impart knowledge or skills to individuals, church leaders, and health care students and professionals involved in or interested in health and health care issues. Included in this approach are organizations that provide information on ecological and public policy issues as well as organizations that provide individuals with information regarding specific illnesses or conditions.

Support and Advocacy

Advocacy and support ministries are grounded first in a loving, serving fellowship—a community of believers that values persons at all stages and seasons of life. Advocacy programs seek to collect resources and raise awareness to promote the inclusion of groups marginalized by virtue of disease or disability, race, age, sex, or socioeconomic status. They do not engage in direct health care. Such programs work in the public arena to influence social, economic, and/or political policy to ensure the fair allocation of health resources and adequate access and response of the health care system to their constituent group.

Support ministries offer association with health care professionals, patients, and church members alike who uphold one another in confidentiality and foster mutual understanding, empathy, and empowerment, both in a broad and in a specific sense. What distinguishes these ministries from educational ministries are their focus on consciousness raising about the needs of particular groups, their compassion, and their caring dimension, encapsulating the pastoral aspect of ministry.

Direct Health Care

Direct health care ministry delivers patient care that embraces prevention and wellness initiatives of public health, diagnostic, intervention, and/or treatment modalities to individual or group clients. The orientation of these services may be either the promotion of wellness or the prevention of sickness. Mental and physical health are included within this definition, as are the concepts of wholistic and integrated health care.

This chapter began with the question How can we discern authentic health and healing ministries? As society at large has become more open to complementary health care practices and has embraced spirituality, prayer, and "faith" as vehicles of healing, the church has a unique opportunity to reclaim its place in moving people toward health and wholeness. The challenge for faith communities is not to retreat into safe havens of orthodoxy concerning healing practice but to allow the winds of the Spirit to fill them with new openness to forms and methods. However, this does not mean we are rudderless. The Christian church, for example, as discussed, has created study and research bodies to wrestle with these questions as well as ecclesiastical groups such as presbyteries, the Anglican Lambeth Conferences, and the writing of great scholars. For the church, though, the most important task is seeing health ministries as reflective of Christ's love, compassion, and inclusion of all God's people. Where Christ is, there is authentic healing.

4

Devotional, Sacramental, and Liturgical Practices

For many people health ministries equal the liturgical healing ministries of the church. Although four areas have been discussed as collectively defining the breadth of health ministries, the first category of the devotional/sacramental/liturgical may be where most churches begin. At the foundation of liturgical healing ministry is a theology that embodies and promotes wholistic health. Its basis is the knowledge that God is the source of all healing. God's power and presence can heal and sustain in the midst of sickness and suffering and provide assurance that even in the face of sin, which may result in sickness, God is with us in our suffering, the "wounded healer."[1]

WORSHIP SERVICES

Healing liturgies are frequently special services that take place outside the context of weekly worship. Nevertheless, the traditional Sunday morning service can be an occasion for promoting spiritual and emotional well-being. This is not to discount special worship experiences using such rituals as the laying on of hands and anointing with oil. Such practices have ancient roots within the Christian tradition, as discussed in chapter 1. But neither should healing through liturgical means be relegated solely to services conducted outside the routine worship life of the community. Rather, concern for the well-being of the community and its members should be incorporated into the ongoing worship life of the congregation.

Pentecost and Christmas highlight key moments in the story of God's people. Other observances, such as All Saints' Day and specific saints' days, are means of remembering and celebrating the lives and work of Christians throughout history. Church observance of anniversaries, weddings, birthdays, and funerals focuses attention on ways in which God is present in the daily as well as the critical times of life. The worship life of the local congregation can touch the full range of emotional and spiritual situations in which church members find themselves. It offers a wide range of possible sustenance and healing through liturgical means.

Despite the importance of healing in regular worship, it is appropriate to have public healing services, though certain precautions against abuse should be observed. The Church of England Archbishops' Report of 1958 is severely critical of public healing services where indiscriminate promises of healing are offered.[2] The dangers include an emphasis in worship on receiving instead of offering; the lack of sufficient preparation; and a failure to recognize the highly emotional component of psychogenic cases and a despair if healing does not take place. Previously noted reservations about faith healing might apply to these criticisms of public healing services.

In some traditions, public healing services are centered in the sacraments. In other more charismatic traditions, the emphasis is on the Holy Spirit's gift of healing or the ministry of deliverance as discussed later in this chapter. A number of pastors find a place for public healing services. "For congregations which have been trained to be a healing community such services provide an experience which is of benefit both corporately and individually."[3] Maddocks suggests that these services have three parts: ministry of the Word; the prayers; and the ministration when the people who wish healing for themselves or someone else come to the altar rail. The Guild of St. Raphael in the United Kingdom has suggested guidelines for specific services: (1) a regular weekday healing service or one after Sunday worship; (2) the use of a smaller worship area or side chapel; (3) the celebration of the eucharist after the intercessions in the service; (4) inclusion of time for people to pray aloud with special needs or concerns; (5) the laying on of hands by the priest, assisted by laypeople; (6) the mention in prayers of specific people; (7) the inclusion of occasional sacramental confession and anointing when appropriate; (8) the avoidance of a service that could be misconstrued as an "exorcism" since it should not be part of public worship; and (9) the provision of counseling afterward.[4]

In addition to public healing services, churches offer prayers, rites, or scriptures especially for those who are sick. These practices have early roots in the life of Israel. The lamentation psalms together with the penitential psalms were used in the liturgy of the cult of the Covenant and its traditions. The individual lament was composed of invocation, lamentation, supplication, motivation, and thanksgiving; its purpose was to give insight into the inner feeling and distress of a sick person. Both the lamentation and the penitential psalms show the link between the worshiping community and the isolated sick person.[5] In many denominational books of worship there are prayers for the sick and dying and their families. A Roman Catholic alternative services book has a service for midlife transition.[6] Other sources have a rite for the removal of life-support systems and for healing after an abortion.[7] There are, of course, special prayers offered for the sick. In the Anglican tradition the first words upon entering the house of a sick person are, "Peace be to this house and to all that dwell in it."[8] Health cannot flourish where bad relationships exist, so invoking this peace is very important.

THE PRACTICE OF PRAYER

Part of the liturgical health ministries is the practice of prayer both individually and collectively; as we saturate ourselves in prayer, we may experience the mystical.[9] Prayer is no magic rite, but can equip us to face problems; it is as essential to our well-being as food and water. It provides no substitute for penicillin or physical therapy, but can bring a change of heart, which medicine alone cannot achieve. "Devote yourselves to prayer," Paul told the Corinthians (1 Cor. 7:5). "Whatever you ask for in prayer with faith, you will receive," Jesus promises (Matt. 21:22).

In the early church, the elders did not simply come to visit but to pray and to encourage others to pray for healing. An important component of prayer is confession and then the removal of guilt and resentment by receiving God's pardon. This clears the way for the inner healing of the person *vis medicatrix naturae*. Confession opens the way for the deeper forces of evil to be confronted and healing to occur.

Types of Prayer

Prayers should begin in silence, in the heart where we listen to God. Prayer has many parts. Prayer is not only petition but also silent adoration where we learn to listen to the voice of God. "Be still and know that I am God."[10] Meditation, which is a form of prayer, is the mind at rest. In a world where relaxation and reflection are rare, it is essential to set aside time for silence and meditation. Silence and meditation have a part in both preventing disease and restoring us to health because they raise our level of awareness. When the mind is still, it can begin to know God. For those experienced in meditation, the longer the silences, the deeper the communion with God. Sometimes the use of a scripture passage or a theme or symbol can center the mind.

The attitude of prayer should be one of relaxation so that we can let God's power surge through us. This creates a sense of expectancy that God's power and peace will fill us. We are trying to put ourselves in alignment with God, to put ourselves in God's presence, so that our knowledge of God and God's purposes for us and the world may grow.

Another aspect of prayer is intercession for others, which should be coupled with works on their behalf.[11] Continuing to pray for others is important, even if we do not see any results, using Jesus as our teacher (Luke 11:5–10; 18:1–14). It is possible that if someone we are praying for dies, that may be God's best answer as God calls that person "home." Our only legitimate prayer for healing is, "Thy will be done," rather than, "If it be God's will," as if there is doubt that God desires healing, though it may be in the sense of ultimate healing in eternity.[12] Corporate prayer may speed recovery and promote healthy attitudes in those praying; we place ourselves in God's service when we pray for someone else. William Temple said that the church is the only organization that exists for the benefit of the outsider, so prayer groups need to be looking outward to community needs.[13] In prayer we draw closer to the Holy Spirit who intercedes for us even when we cannot articulate our needs (Rom. 8:26–27). Prayer brings us into accord with God's will, promoting trust and obedience to God as well as thanksgiving for all God has done.

Some have raised the question whether one's prayers should be for healing of a specific ailment or problem or a more general request. John Fitzpatrick relates the case of a man who tried for years to give up smoking. He prayed that God would take away his craving for tobacco. He was successful only when he recognized his smoking was tied to rebellion against his father. When he healed the relationship with his father, he stopped smoking.[14] His prayers needed to be about understanding the reason for his addiction, which was his relationship with his father, not simply asking God to remove his craving for tobacco. (This illustration does not, however, address the multidimensional nature of addiction.)

Petitionary prayer may lead us to a deeper relationship with God where God's will is our deepest desire (Matt. 26:39). When we come in stark need, our concentration is heightened. God always hears our petitions but does not automatically grant them. However, when God's Spirit infuses us, our outlook can be transformed.

The Results of Prayer

In discussing the results of prayer it may be instructive to return to some of the earlier material on the scientific studies referenced by Larson and

Dossey. For many Christians discussing prayer's results in scientific terms may seem off-putting, as most people refer to prayer's "results" in subjective terms.

Prayer's Impact on Heart Patients. *The Faith Factor,* cited earlier, highlights studies that show positive outcomes with specific illnesses. A 1988 study written up by R. B. Byrd in the *Southern Medical Journal* profiled the effect of intercessory prayer for ten months on 393 patients in a large county hospital in San Francisco. Its conclusion was that "patients admitted to a coronary care unit in a large county hospital who received intercessory prayer on their behalf" by select intercessors to the Judeo-Christian God "had fewer life-threatening events and complications after entering into the study than the control group."[15]

Effectiveness of Different Types of Prayer. Dossey explores different types of prayer to introduce the discussion about which kind may be most effective. When we pray, we should pay attention to the unconscious mind. We can accomplish this to a large extent by getting in touch with our dreams. We can pray while we are dreaming. Dreams and prayer may come together to produce healing. Prayer here is defined as an "urge towards oneness," unity, and wholeness.[16] He points to the Spindrift organization experiments in Salem, Oregon, which seem to confirm that nondirect prayer is best, but Dossey concludes that one method of prayer should not be favored over another. We should not instruct God by our prayers, as they should be invitations rather than specific requests. Open-ended prayers requesting only that "thy will be done" appear to be significantly more effective than directed prayer for a specific outcome. However, we should not capture this into a "formula" because other illustrations of imagery and visualization are very specific and also bring healing.[17]

The value of studies, especially by Spindrift, is their demonstration that prayer is effective.[18] There is no specific formula shown to be the best, but being true to one's spirituality and letting go are important. Dossey warns against those who practice formulas like "right-thinking" since they blame failure on the patient and not the formula. Silence and stillness, as the great saints have testified, may be the best way of knowing God's presence. He suggests that relaxation and attention training may be helpful in adopting a really prayerful attitude. Furthermore, nondirected prayer may be the best guard against understanding God as our errand boy. Ann and Barry Ulanov, professors at Union Theological Seminary in New York City, refer to this thinking as seeing God as the "big prayer jukebox." In this model we see our prayers like coins put into the jukebox and we select a specific tune. However, we quickly discover the jukebox is not always playing the tune we expect.[19]

Dossey's data include those who pray and those for whom prayers are offered. As in *The Faith Factor* studies, he cites as noteworthy the "randomized, double-blind Byrd experiment in which neither the patients, nurses, nor doctors knew" which of 200 out of 400 patients admitted to the coronary unit received prayer. While Byrd's study was initially enthusiastically embraced, it soon came under fire from the scientific community for a number of reasons, including questions about "prayer strategies." But Dossey lauds Byrd nevertheless for his "courage" in conducting the study in the modern medical environment.[20]

Dossey's main objective in faulting these early studies is that the effectiveness of prayer might better be measured using nonhuman living systems, with fewer variables to complicate the results. He cites PEAR's measurements of "the actions of the consciousness" as a model of cutting edge methodology.[21]

Prayer's Effect on "Nonhuman Studies." Among the studies Dossey cites, he gives the strongest credence to the PEAR Institute and the Benor studies because of their scientific validity in substantiating the power of prayer to heal. Daniel Benor, an American psychiatrist working in England, collected 131 studies of "spiritual healing" mostly in nonhuman fungus cultures.[22] He defined "spiritual healing" as "the intentional influence of one or more people upon another living system without utilizing known physical means of intervention." Spiritual here is defined as anything nonphysical that reinforces what we said earlier about the nebulous definitions given to the word "spiritual."

There were several conclusions from this study. The first is that "if genetic mutations can be influenced by the conscious efforts of others, as in one of the above studies, then genes cannot be the absolute controllers they are represented to be." The mind can cause bad genes to mutate into good ones. What is most important is that "spiritual healing can be completely independent of the 'psychology' of the subject."[23] However, Dossey's most interesting conclusion of all is buried at the end of this section: "It appears that double-blind studies can sometimes be steered in directions that correspond to the thoughts and attitudes of the experimenters. This might shed light on why skeptical experimenters appear unable to replicate the findings of believers, and why 'true believers' seem more able to produce positive results."[24]

Theologians Look at Prayer's Effect. Moving from the scientific to the theological perspective on prayer, Leslie Weatherhead raises one of the central questions concerning the result of prayer: What is the point of intercession for the sick when the physical condition of the patient does not change? Weatherhead uses the black plague as an example of why God did not directly intervene to save people. He argues that if God had saved everyone, then medical science would not have found a cure for the plague.[25] (This seems like a rather unusual line of argument since even if some prayers for those dying of the plague were answered, a cure could still have been discovered.)

However, Weatherhead is right that we should continue praying not because our prayers are successful or unsuccessful but because we are commanded to pray for the sick. Christians pray because we are bidden to, not because we understand how prayer works. Prayer should be both private and corporate, done in confidence rather than doubt, with consistency and faith. Prayer groups are best formed by one-on-one invitations, not general announcements. The effectiveness of intercession is not in direct relation to the numbers involved; hundreds of people praying are not necessary for an ill person to recover.[26] Jesus never drew a correlation between healing and the number of people praying. It may be the case, however, that a patient is empowered by knowing that many people are praying for her—defeat, despair, and pessimism can be exchanged for courage and the will to live.

What are the various effects of prayer? Our prayers cannot make God love us more or deepen God's desire for our health, but they reflect thanksgiving for God's goodness and love for us. God will show us when we pray where we have gone wrong and what changes are necessary in our lives. Prayer shows our dependence upon God; with God all things are possible.

The difficulty with understanding the relationship between prayer and healing is that it again raises the question of the relationship between sin and sickness.[27] This question is most poignant when the patient prayed for either continues in a painful illness or dies. Was there a spiritual defect in the person praying or being prayed for that occasioned this resistance to healing?

David Watson, the great British evangelist and preacher, recounts his own unsuccessful, heroic struggle against cancer. He had a powerful healing ministry throughout the United Kingdom where many had been healed. He repeatedly reviewed events in his life to discover what might be blocking his healing. No matter how he prayed or what he did or whom he forgave, physical healing never took place. The events had a strong impact on those involved in his ministry as they realized physical healing does not always take place. He died with full confirmation that God was in control and that he need fear no evil.[28]

In wrestling with the problem of why some are healed and others are not, our first question should not be why the person is sick or whether we should pray for healing, but what gesture of solidarity we can offer with the one who is suffering. As Paul wrote in Colossians 1:24, "I am now rejoicing in my sufferings for your sake, and in my flesh I am completing what is lacking in Christ's afflictions for the sake of his body, that is, the church."

As central as prayer is to any healing ministry, however, healing agents should not be reduced solely to prayer or faith. Medicine, physicians, and other persons may be instruments of healing. Jesus used numerous means for healing—touch, a command, physical agents, the following of instructions, prayer, and/or faith. Many people get well without any of these agents or remain sick even with prayer, medicine, and the presence of loved ones. No matter what the means, God is the source of all healing. This thought is expressed in the words over Columbia Presbyterian Medical Center: "From on the most high cometh healing."[29] There is one source of healing but different means and results of healing. God uses all means for our healing—prayer, medication, surgery; and our faith in God can work as a means in itself.[30]

If God heals, what is the purpose of medicine and prayer? Both of them have the effect of opening a person to God's healing power, of removing the obstacles to healing. Prayer calls on the healing gifts of the Spirit, which are as real and powerful as any drug. Medicine eliminates the physical barriers inhibiting the body's healing process, while prayer unclogs the pores of the soul, opening one to God's grace.

Medicine differs from prayer in that it can be administered without acknowledging God's power. Prayer, never so. Furthermore, medicine has limited efficacy if the disease is not cured. But prayer is efficacious even if the disease continues to run its course. An inner calm, a lessening of pain, a speedier recovery—all may be the results of prayer. Even if the body is not cured, the spirit may be restored.

THE ADMINISTRATION OF THE SACRAMENTS

Another part of the liturgical health ministries is the administration of sacraments. Sacraments are not given to the sick just to make them feel good but have a power in and of themselves. In the Anglican and Roman Catholic traditions sacraments form part of the healing ministry, making it a much more natural part of the life of the church instead of a separate ministry.

Although the various Christian traditions have not reached consensus on the number of sacraments, the major traditions recognize baptism and Holy Communion. The sacraments are means by which God's grace is offered to a repentant humanity and signs of God's ongoing activity in the world. The sacraments are gifts from God, available to all who accept the new life that God offers in Christ. The different elements of the sacraments are often used interchangeably. For example, laying on of hands and anointing are sometimes used in baptism, healing, and ordination.

The term in the ante-Nicene church for sacrament often was "medicine of life" (*pharmakia*) by which the regenerate life was built up.[31] The sacraments are the means by which the nature of the old order becomes interpenetrated by the power of the Holy Spirit. In one sense the law of cause and effect cannot be traced, but God is the source of their power.

Augustine declared that the sacrament itself was one thing and that the power of the sacrament was another, that is, its essence and its effect are different. This definition is important as we think of the healing nature of the sacraments that may or may not be the case for every individual.[32] The efficacy of the sacraments lies not in the work of the minister but in the conjunction of the divine promises associated with the sacraments that make proclamation necessary; the use of the appointed elements; and the faith of the recipient.

Healing from the sacraments comes as a result of our faith in God, who works through us.[33] Through the regular administration of the sacraments, members of the church community are reminded of the life of grace and obedience to which we are called. The sacraments signify and seal God's power and gifts, which the church uses in healing; they represent forgiveness, reconciliation, and love. They remind us that Christ has given of the Divine Self for all of creation, which is blessed in Christ's name. They reaffirm the believers' dependence upon grace and symbolize hope.

Every object, indeed every event, has the potential to be sacramental. A sacrament is an outward sign and portent of a spiritual reality. The common elements of everyday life such as bread and wine become holy when infused with the Holy Spirit. This holiness is made real by the actions of human beings who dedicate themselves to God. God created the world and saw that it was good. The sacraments remind us of the holiness of all creation. When we have been fully immersed in the sacramental reality of common life, we will be able to sense the divine presence in all of life's circumstances. God's presence is manifested through the sacraments. God's created order is progressive and not static. God's work, which is already good, may become more productive and highly developed.

Our new creation points to the greatness of the transformation brought by the sacraments.[34] They become the contact with the vitality of life in God. The physical effect of partaking of the sacraments is an unbroken communion with God. Attempts for scientific explanations of the sacraments are difficult. However, it is true that the scientific community is recognizing that we can no longer draw sharp lines between spirit and matter.

The Eucharist

The various names for the eucharist—the Lord's Supper, Holy Communion, the Mass—express different meanings. Our analysis is from the perspective of the Protestant church in the United States and the Church of England rather than the Roman Catholic Church, so the term "Mass" will not be used.

Communion calls to remembrance the gift of forgiveness and renewal through Christ's death. It is both a memorial to Christ's sacrifice and an entrance into eternal life. In partaking of communion, we are reminded that all that we eat and drink has a sacramental quality, that the breaking of bread is a sign of hospitality. The worshiping community is reminded that we are like a broken body, shedding blood. We are taken apart, we are sick and in pain, we need healing; yet the sacrament tangibly shows us God's sign, God's nourishment, God's gift of life and health. No matter how broken we are, Christ renews us. The fruit of the earth is a source of healing; the vision in Revelation 22:2—"the leaves of the tree are for the healing of the nations"—captures this image.

The link between the eucharist and healing is not clearly reflected in the Synoptic Gospels. However, in the Corinthian church, a failure to partake correctly of the bread and wine as the body of Christ could lead to ill health and death (1 Cor. 11:27–30). The link of the eucharist to one's spiritual and physical health in the early church was discussed in chapter 1. Every eucharist proclaims the present reality of the beginning of the reign of God. Healing of unsatisfactory relationships can take place through the Lord's Supper. Here we receive forgiveness for what we have done to others. In the eucharist, through Christ, we find an openness to the past and to the present, to heaven and to the world. It is the anticipatory celebration of a healed creation, foreshadowing the coming of God's reign.[36] Communion becomes a corporate act with those in the church—removing our sense of isolation. When they take communion to people who are homebound, many pastors fail to reflect on its healing dimension; how much richer this sacrament could be, especially when the pastor is accompanied by one or two elders who represent the communion with the saints.[37]

Baptism

As one of the two sacraments accepted in all Christian traditions, baptism may reflect a healing dimension. In baptism, water as a cleansing agent is a symbol of the death of the old personality and resurrection of the soul into new life. Baptism is the initial healing sacrament as it brings the person symbolically through death and isolation into the community of believers. Because of its communal nature and pledge by the congregation to bring the child up in the "nurture and admonition" of God, in many traditions there are no godparents; the covenant community assumes this function.

In baptism, one is "born anew" into Christ's family. Baptism is a sign of new life and health, God's gifts, given with water. In John's apocalyptic vision, the river of the water of life flowing from the throne of God and of the Lamb is for healing.[38] "Then the angel showed me the river of the water of life, bright as crystal, flowing from the throne of God and of the Lamb" (Rev. 22:1). Baptism historically has included, in many churches, the anointing with oil (a sign of the outpouring of the Holy Spirit) and the laying on of hands (a sign of God's own touch). Throughout life, every act of worship, such as anointing, laying on of hands, or participating in the baptism of another child of God, is an opportunity to reaffirm, and be thankful for, one's own baptismal promises. It calls for the promise of support from the community of believers.

According to Maddocks, baptism has been called the primary healing sacrament because it sets into motion the healing of our birth experience. For patristic Father Hilary, baptism makes us the recipient of God's Spirit and immune from death, in addition to obliterating our sins. For Ambrose (ca. 339–97), it provides rebirth.[39] The central symbol for the work of Christ was reconciliation, which occurs when we receive forgiveness for our sins. Even in the Roman Catholic Church penance is now seen as the renewal of baptismal grace and therefore as a reconciling act with God and the church.[40] Unfortunately, for many contemporary Christians baptism has lost much of its power compared to its practice in the ante-Nicene church: "it is possible for professing Christians to set more store by the vaccination of their babies than by their Baptism."[41]

LITURGICAL PRACTICES

The sacraments are important in healing, but general liturgical practices are also worthy of note. Worship includes not only sacraments but various rites as well that constitute an important part of praising and glorifying God and help us to move toward wholeness.

The Rite of Healing

Since many traditions do not accept the sacrament of healing but use some of its elements, it is referred to here as a rite. Several elements constitute this rite of healing—laying on of hands, anointing, absolution, and celebration of the eucharist. Not all elements are used on every occasion or by every denomination. The references here are for principal use in the Anglican tradition. An extensive discussion of the history of this rite was covered in chapter 1. Even in the Church of England the instructions and parts of this service, eventually called "Ministry to the Sick," were hotly debated, and the service was not included in the *Alternative Services Book* but is a separate booklet.[42] Three separate items concerning a ministry of healing were to be considered: services for use with the sick; a form for the "Reconciliation of a Penitent"; and the "Blessing of the Oils." There has been an increased use of various elements of this rite in Protestant healing services, especially the practice of anointing by Protestant hospital chaplains.[43]

The Laying On of Hands. There are theological and psychological roots to the practice of the laying on of hands. Theologically, it is an act of adoption, so it has become the outward sign of commissioning people to ministry. In the healing ministry, it draws us into the body of Christ so that we may receive Christ's healing power. Psychologically, love is expressed by touch. Touch has deep spiritual significance. It is God's hand that touches the person through another.[44] Many consider touch an integral part of patient care. It can be of benefit physically, psychologically, and socially; hence using touch in Christ's healing ministry is a natural way to minister to others.[45]

The laying on of hands reflects how we can be a channel of God's power; it is Christ's touching. Sometimes people who receive the laying on of hands testify to sensations of power, heat, light, and tingling. However, the concentration should be on Christ's healing power, not its physical manifestations. Sensitivity to possible negative interpretations of touch in certain cultures is crucial. Touch should be practiced only with permission. Caution over positioning of hands and the use of teams or pairs of ministers would seem reasonable, especially in today's climate of concern about sexual innuendo or harassment that is associated with unwelcome touch.

The practices of the laying on of hands and anointing with oil have their precedence in the Holy Scriptures. "They will lay their hands on the sick" (Mark 16:18); in the Hebrew Scriptures touch was not used as a method of healing. The only related practice was the stretching out of one's hands over the children's bodies by Elijah (1 Kings 17:21–22) and Elisha (2 Kings 4:32–34). The laying on of hands was associated with the idea of designating a person for a specific purpose for God. This is an extension of the idea that through God's hand, God's power is made known.

There are two different forms of imposition of hands in the Hebrew. One is *samak*, meaning "to lean" or "rest upon." This imposition of hands signifies the transference of power used in Numbers 27:18, 23 for the commissioning of Joshua as Moses' substitute. The other words *sim* and *shit*, meaning "putting" and "placing," are used in the sense of blessing and healing, for example, the blessing Jacob gave to (literally, put on) his sons (Gen. 48:14).

Jesus used touch for both blessing and healing. Christ touched and blessed the children. The Gospel texts use the plural for Jesus' laying on of hands, *epitheis tas cheiras*. In Mark's Gospel the imposition of hands is commended to the apostles as a means of healing by Christ (Mark 16:18). In the Church of England the laying on of hands is witnessed in confirmation, in the Ordinal, and in the earlier ceremony of touching for the King's Evil.[46] In Acts, touch was used by the disciples, for example, Ananias's laying on of hands to cure Saul's blindness (Acts 9:17–19), and Paul's healing Publius's father from a fever (Acts 28:7–10). Other instances of touch are mentioned in Acts 3:7; 14:19–20; 19:11; and 20:10.

After the time of the apostles, the laying on of hands was formalized and practiced widely. The laying on of hands had three associations: (1) the symbol of contact with the Holy Spirit; (2) a reminder of the nature of God, who desires the wholeness of all people; and (3) the fulfillment of prayer.[47] The subsequent liturgical history of the imposition of hands was most evident in the rites of ordination and baptism.

The laying on of hands is not considered a formal ministry but a sign of identification with another person. In the Anglican tradition there are a number of instructions about the laying on of hands, some of which form the basis of the following exposition. This practice is less formal in contrast to anointing, which is considered a somewhat weightier ministry. A sick person may request anointing, but if the request is made frequently or the complaint is something trivial, the pastor will then advise the inappropriateness of anointing. The form of words for anointing may vary but is to address the whole person.

The laying on of hands is always linked with prayer. There is a "straight line" from apostolic practice to our own day but without a certainty of physical healing. The prayers offered should direct the sick person's attention to God because the tendency is often to become morbidly introspective. Care should be taken neither to arouse false expectations nor to suggest impending death while recognizing that God's understanding of true wholeness is far greater than ours.

There may also be different prayers for someone who is dying, and the forehead may be marked with the sign of the cross. The dying person should always be addressed as if he or she can hear you and should never be discussed as if he or she was not present. However, simply entrusting to God or letting go of a loved person could be appropriate. The prayers that are used vary greatly, but all are based on the belief that God wants to heal us.

In the Church of England healing rites are often part of the regular worship service. The sermon, explanation, intercessions, penitence, laying on of hands and anointing, canticle, creed, prayers, the Te Deum, a psalm, and a blessing become part of morning or evening prayers.[48] There is no mention of exorcism as part of the service. Of course, the heart of the service for the sick is communion since it is a weekly occurrence within the life of the Anglican Church.

Laying on of hands and anointing were to be done after communion in the Anglican tradition so that those who wanted it could remain at the rail or go to a side chapel.[49] If the sick person is unable to receive communion, a provision for a "spiritual communion" is set forth in Note 8 of the worship service. Partaking by homebound persons from the parish communion was considered an important practice to symbolize the connection with the community.[50]

Preparation of the sick person for this rite was considered very important and beforehand involved several pastoral visits. The priest's *vade mecum* contained scriptural lessons and prayers, which were used to prepare the patient. There are three qualifications for the fruitful reception of this rite: faith, repentance, and charity. Unction is a remedial rather than an absolving rite, according to Charles Harris.[51]

The anointing itself is a simple service: an anointing with oil on the forehead with the sign of the cross, together with a prayer of anointing. The oil is blessed and used, and then removed from the sick person's forehead with a piece of cloth, which is subsequently burned. A form for the "Blessing of the Oils" was defeated but later included in the appendix. Also the form for the "Reconciliation of a Penitent" was not included in the service because of the controversial words "I absolve you" instead of "you are absolved." No provision for exorcism was included.[52]

In summary, the rite of healing is used for those who have declared their need in advance and been prepared for this ministry. It is a corporate ministry where the congregation joins in the prayers for the people. There is also allowance in more charismatic traditions for laying on of hands during the intercessory prayers by members of the congregation. In these services links are made between confession and healing, which are followed by the Peace as an assurance of the corporate undergirding of sick persons.

It is important to keep the practice of the rite of healing within the church because solo ministers are open to many dangers. Who should administer anointing and the laying on of hands is a subject for much discussion. Some people believe that only ordained clergy and people with the gift of healing should practice anointing. It is clear that people who practice the laying on of hands should be recognized by the church and set apart in some way. This can best be done by recognizing the sacramental aspects of this ministry and understanding its practice by those who are validated to serve the sacraments. The power of the rite of healing, as the eucharist, rests in the corporate nature of these rites—we are joined with one another as well as with Christ.

The Ministry of Deliverance

The last liturgical practice of the church to be examined is that of exorcism—a barely understood and rarely practiced rite. Here it is designated as a rite, not a sacrament, a legitimate practice in *rare* cases as part of a health ministry. The broader category under which exorcism falls is the ministry of deliverance. What does the ministry of deliverance have to do with the healing ministry of the church? Should we address this topic at all? Many popular charismatic healers have built a large part of their healing ministries on the practice of deliverance. Most Protestant church members associate exorcism with fringe groups or former times when people were burned as witches; surprisingly enough, demon possession continues to be reported today.

Since the popularity of John Wimber in the United States and the United Kingdom, it has become even more important to understand this phenomenon. Wimber was an evangelist with a worldwide healing ministry who had a large following on both continents. As a visiting professor at Fuller Theological Seminary in Pasadena, California, in 1987, I was asked to teach on the role of the church in healing in the wake of the great controversy over the courses on healing taught by Wimber and Peter Wagner (a professor at the School of World Religions at Fuller Seminary). Exorcisms and miraculous healings were performed in their classroom. The question was not only about the appropriateness of these events in general, but most especially in a theological seminary.[53]

In my thirty years as an ordained minister, I have had only three specific requests for an exorcism. The first one was in Brazil in 1962, when my infant son was diagnosed by a superstitious neighbor as having an evil spirit.[54] The second request was by a secretary working in the Interchurch Center in New York City in the 1970s. She had been using Ouija boards and was into occult practices prior to her conversion to Christianity. (I referred her to the One Flock Charismatic group in New York City.) The third case was of a woman in Washington, D.C., who believed she was possessed by multiple spirits. (I referred her to a Jesuit priest at

Georgetown University.) Also in the 1970s when I was a chaplain at Columbia University, I participated in "deprogramming" several students who had become involved in the occult, witchcraft, Satanism, and sect and cult groups.

Christian Scriptures' Perspectives on Casting Out Demons.
Assessing the appropriateness of exorcism and a ministry of deliverance as part of a health ministry requires a review of the material in the Christian Scriptures on this subject. Jesus described his ministry in the coming of the realm of God as confronting Satan. The devil tried to tempt him in the wilderness and to amass his powers at the time of Christ's crucifixion (John 14:30; Luke 22:53), but Jesus saw Satan falling from heaven, overcome by God's power (Luke 10:18).[55] Since the irrationality of sickness may reflect that Satan has control of this world, a patient may need spiritual as well as physical and psychological treatment. However, this is different from exorcising demons.

Jesus diagnosed possession as possible when extraordinary strength and disregard for pain were present (Mark 5:3). In three stories the demoniacs were disturbed when confronted by Jesus (Mark 1:24; 5:7; 9:20). Of course, Jesus used his own name when calling forth the demons. Jesus performed exorcisms but limited them to the rare cases where they were necessary.

There are a number of biblical accounts of exorcisms. Mary Magdalene had to be cleansed of seven devils. After the resurrection the followers of Jesus not only challenged the rule of Satan but also cast out devils (Mark 16:17; Acts 5:16; 19:12–20). Demon possession, however, was only one of many diagnoses of illness; people were cured of every kind of illness (Matt. 4:24).

Early Church Views of Demon Possession.
According to patristic scholar Evelyn Frost, the ante-Nicene church centered its healing ministry on confrontation with evil. It saw the twofold task of Christian healing as dealing with ontological evil and its symptoms. The ancient methods of combating evil in the ante-Nicene church were twofold: absolution and exorcism. These were considered means of grace and preparation for the two great sacraments, eucharist and baptism. The main purpose of exorcism was for the Holy Spirit to possess the entire personality.

The matter of demon possession raises the whole question about the nature of evil: Is it personal or impersonal?[56] Is there a personal devil who can possess people? Is evil an objective, ontological reality, or does evil exist only when people commit sinful acts? The early church believed in personal, objective evil; hence exorcism was necessary. The best word on the subject may be that of C. S. Lewis: "There are two equal and opposite errors into which our race can fall about devils. One is to disbelieve in their existence; the other is to believe, and to feel an excessive and unhealthy interest in them. They themselves are equally pleased by both errors."[57]

Charismatic Groups Rediscover Exorcism. The rediscovery of exorcism has been mainly among Pentecostal and charismatic groups under the name of the ministry of deliverance. Their theology is based on being Spirit filled. This can happen only by a total deliverance from spirits that oppress or possess. Although we applaud the centrality of the Holy Spirit in their theology, historical safeguards against the possible abuses of a deliverance ministry may be absent.

Many charismatic groups believe that dominion over spirits is possible only through the victory of Jesus at Calvary (John 12:31; 16:11). Satan is a defeated enemy and has no rights or authority over a believer—Satan is there only by deception. The church as the body of Christ has authority to release people but needs to be taught to undertake this ministry (Matt. 10:1; Mark 3:14–15; 6:13; Luke 9:1–2; 10:17). In practice, the deliverance is performed by the evangelist/healer, who is believed to possess the gift of discernment in language reminiscent of Ephesians 6:10–18 and Luke 11:14–28. The believer's authority in these spiritual realms is stressed; physical symptoms often accompany these acts of exorcism. However, the charismatic healers acknowledge that deliverance may not be permanent.

Some practitioners of deliverance describe a threefold movement of the stages of demonic control: (1) *oppression* occurs in the realm of the mind, where people are influenced to disbelieve God's Word and live worldly lives (Eph. 2:1–3); (2) *obsession* develops when Satan draws a person into deeper subjection—the person no longer desires freedom; and (3) *possession* takes place when Satan has assumed control over one or more areas of a person's body, mind, or spirit. Various orders of demons and personality disturbances and physical illnesses are associated with possession, among them: blind spirits, deaf spirits, deception, seduction, jealousy, lies, insanity, addictions, and cancers. Indeed the harboring of wrong attitudes—anger, bitterness, hatred, and/or unforgiveness—opens a person to oppression if not possession by a controlling spirit.

These practitioners often operate from an uncritical view of demon possession. As some scholars have pointed out, they do not acknowledge psychological insights regarding spirits and possession. If people are possessed, what is possessing them? Are there evil spirit entities from outside that infect people, or are they deep, unhealed areas of the unconscious mind that manifest themselves in strange ways?

Contemporary Views of Demon Possession. Michael Welker, professor of systematic theology in Heidelberg, Germany, argues that demon possession is real, not some antiquated science translated by writers of the Christian Scriptures. "Are not demons products of unbelief and superstition who in the sober, realistic, enlightened, scientific view of the world disappear like fog in the sunlight?" Welker asks. His response is an emphatic "No." Where we find "stabilized and stubbornly defended" suffering in the world today, we find demon possession. Their names might be different from those we encounter in the accounts of Mark 1:26; 9:17–18; and Luke 4:35. In the twentieth century, Welker says, we might recognize demon possession in addiction, greed, ecological ruin, and the debt politics of developing nations. Jesus Christ, bearer of the Holy Spirit, is the liberator from all distress, captivity, and hopelessness and the restorer of coherent and peaceful ways.[58]

Welker's definition of demon possession is quite different from the strict definitions applied by church commissions on exorcism. He tends to equate sin and demon possession and collapse the various nuances of related phenomena as described in the Church of England Report. Although we cannot explain away all possession in the Christian Scriptures as simply mental illness, neither can we automatically "baptize" various manifestations of sin as demon possession.

Many contemporary Christians see the accounts in the Christian Scriptures of exorcism as ways of explaining disease that reflect superstitions of a long-past world. Keir Howard takes the point of view that they were metaphors for psychological disturbances.[59] No demon of lust was expelled from the adulterous woman or from the incestuous people of Corinth. No demon of avarice was expelled from Zacchaeus. Relatively speaking, there were few exorcisms among Christ's forty healing miracles.

Exorcism Study Group Report. One of the best resources on the subject of exorcism was prepared by the Church of England Christian Exorcism Study Group. The findings of this study group are not only applicable to the Anglican Church but can help U.S. churches better understand this phenomenon. This group generated a comprehensive study and has helped to train those who advise Anglican bishops in this area. Interestingly enough, no rite of exorcism is included in this document. However, in the Church of Wales Prayer Book the ministry of healing includes the ministry of deliverance.[60] The statement accompanying its inclusion is fascinating:

> Healing is part of the total ministry of the Church: prayer and sacraments are its foundations. As we administer Christ's healing we need always to be aware of the differing levels of illness: first the illness itself, secondly the anxieties and fears that may underlie

or precipitate it. On occasion it is possible to identify a third and deeper level in which we realize that "we are not contending against flesh and blood, but against the principalities, against the powers, against the world rulers of this present darkness, against the spiritual hosts of wickedness in the heavenly places [Ephesians 6:12]."[61]

The American Episcopal Church mentions exorcism in its 1994 *Book of Occasional Services*, affirming the bishop as the one who determines whether it is needed, who will perform it, and rites used.[62]

The Anglican Church Study Group begins by defining terms. Exorcism is "the spiritual cleansing of a place which is believed to be infested by the demoniac, but most usually 'a specific act of binding and releasing, performed on a person who is believed to be possessed by a non-human malevolent spirit.'"[63] This report discusses the underlying causes of possession: an unrepentant life of sin; occultism; deliberate subjection to a satanic cult; occultism in the family; or bargains with the devil. A person is demon possessed if he wills to do only evil and can no longer control his impulses; there is masochistic pleasure in any hurt committed to his body or to others. There will be physical signs, such as a bilious complexion and a wasting away of the body. Any conversation on Christian subjects with possessed persons occasions screaming, cursing, raving, and violent behavior on their part. There are many different reactions to the exorcist when the demon is doing everything to avoid being exorcised. After reading the vivid descriptions of these possessed people and the accompanying exorcism, there is no way to confuse them with typical psychotic episodes. The vile words, foaming at the mouth, violent behavior, and obsession with evil are terrifying manifestations.

This report also defines the freeing of possessed people as deliverance. Deliverance "is about freeing people from the bondage of Satan," which may not require a formal exorcism with sacramental rites but is accomplished by "slaying in the spirit."[64] The most frequent cause of appeal to the Exorcism Study Group for help is poltergeist disturbances,[65] which consist of moving objects, sounds, breaking of objects, cold spots, and sounds of music. These occurrences, I might add, have been reported in one of the early-nineteenth-century faculty houses at Princeton Theological Seminary.

Guidelines are offered by the commission for counselors who are faced with a specific case of suspected possession or satanic involvement. They stress the importance of the interview, diagnosis, preparatory prayer, consultation with the bishop and the medical profession, and method and forms of service for exorcism. This ministry must be firmly under the discipline of the church. Most churches agree that following an exorcism, there should be a prayer of blessing and committal to Christ in everyday life.[66] In balance, in the parishes of the Church of England "possession" is always the last diagnosis to be made when all else has been exhausted. Bishop Maddocks, involved in the healing ministry for forty years, stated he had performed only two exorcisms during all those years.[67]

Concrete steps are outlined for a priest/pastor to follow when demon possession is suspected. First, write a detailed case history in order to clearly assess the case and not prejudge it. Second, pray inwardly for the person. Third, keep calm, and remember the purpose is to bring healing; do not allow the strange and frightening manifestations to overwhelm you. Fourth, investigate the social, family, medical, and spiritual background of all concerned. This may reveal certain cultural predispositions to curses or the abuse of hallucinatory drugs, which could cause visions or fantasies about devils. Fifth, act like a pastor, not a judge. If you do not understand what is happening, be compassionate and supportive. Sixth, use a joint ministry with medical practitioners or psychiatrists whenever possible. It is imperative that exorcists work in close cooperation with medical practitioners. In other words, before a decision that an exorcism is warranted, scientific medicine should make a diagnosis of the patient's condition. Seventh, make the client feel welcome and not judged. However, if there has been involvement with a Ouija board or the occult, a formal renunciation of Satan and acceptance of Christ should take place; one may accept the person while judging the behavior. Eighth, if the case seems straightforward, use prayer, laying on of hands, anointing, and celebration of the eucharist as the means of exorcism rather than following a particular rite of exorcism. Ninth, call for assistance from pastors experienced in this matter in more complex cases and receive permission and blessings from the bishop. Religious houses sometimes are especially equipped to deal with these matters. Tenth, offer after-care for anyone who shows symptoms of possession. It is very important to connect the person with a Christian companion and help the client see this experience as a call to a deeper relationship with Christ.[68] This pastoral after-care is the responsibility not only of the parish priest but also of the whole congregation.[69]

As a pastor goes through the initial stages of assessment, she may determine that ordinary counseling and psychiatric treatments may suffice without the need for exorcism. The sightings of ghosts and place memories where evil spirits are present have been corroborated by trained Anglican priests (for example, the sites of wars, murders, and so forth) but are cases not for exorcism, but for prayers and blessings. Training and discernment to avoid the particular dangers of abuse are crucial. Working in pairs may be extremely important to assist in discernment.

There may be confusion among the various phenomena of the occult, psychic appearances, and demon possession, making an assessment about the need for an exorcism difficult. The psychic is not the same as the occult.[70] Psychics are not necessarily spiritually oriented. The psychic is not innately spiritual but may use his or her gifts in God's service. Psychic powers may be gifts from God but must be used properly. The Bible contains several warnings against psychic phenomena, which are seen as a form of idolatry (see, for example, Lev. 19:31; 20:6; Deut. 18:10–11). These biblical prohibitions refer to an unauthorized and unspiritual manipulation of the psychic.[71]

Other distinctions that need to be drawn are among witchcraft, Satanism, and demon possession. While federal law prohibits satanic organizations, there are not laws against witchcraft groups, which move more freely in society. Satanic groups often recruit teenagers with low self-esteem who are vulnerable and lonely. Witchcraft is generally linked more to those with an affinity to nature whereas Satanism is truly aligned with evil. Even "projections" that become visible may not need exorcism. Perhaps these places of the visions should be blessed and sprinkled with holy water, and a prayer for health and care in the name of Christ offered.

Only after understanding these other phenomena, according to the commission, can we address the subject of possession.[72] Possession may be a case of psychological projection. It may be the natural defenses of the ego against anxiety, conflict, and guilt. These emotions must be eliminated in the ill person before a pastor attempts to practice an exorcism. There are, of course, a wide range of neurotic and personality disorders, including schizophrenia, which have in the past been confused with demon possession.

Exorcisms of Places and Institutions—Social Exorcisms. An interesting category of exorcism that recently has been documented in various books on the healing ministry is exorcism performed on social institutions and buildings. There is a deep need for the healing of social institutions, families, congregations, and nations. The word in the Hebrew Scriptures for healing, *shalom*, connotes this social dimension. The Church of England in the previously mentioned study also cites exorcisms of buildings. A Welsh Anglican priest in October 1997 recounted to me the story of a church that he pastored, which had been the site of one of the battles of the Hundred Years' War (1337–1453 C.E.). A sense of evil and foreboding permeated the church. The membership never grew because people felt a sense of dread upon entering the church. Cold spots were detected, and objects moved. The priest submitted his request for the exorcism of the building, which was reviewed by the local bishop. After an extensive review by the bishop, the need for an exorcism was corroborated. The rite was presided over by the bishop and the priest in the presence of several members of the church. After the exorcism, people who had been unaware that it was performed marked a noted change in the building; the sense of dread was gone, and a welcoming air prevailed.

Other cases of social exorcisms are cited in the United States. Although they are labeled exorcisms, they certainly do not seem to fit into our previous definition of this term. These appear to be cases not of ontological evil but of negativity, unpleasantness, or conflict. One case presented under the rubric of a social exorcism was of a church where the members were relentlessly negative. It was discovered that the former church site had been bought by the state and was covered by a lake, so the old church was literally under water. There was a bitterness associated with this event by the members of the church, even though it had happened years ago. The current pastor, part of a prayer group of clergy, asked the group to pray for the church. Her prayer request was that the waters that had meant drowning and death to the church should be transformed into baptismal water leading to new life. As a symbolic expression of this institutional baptismal renewal, members of the group moved from room to room in the church sprinkling water in each room while asking a blessing. From that time forward, the church members began to change. New members joined, the building was open to Alcoholics Anonymous and other self-help groups, and the pastor noticed a change in her attitude.[73] Were these changes the result of changed attitudes or the rites practiced? What do we think of baptizing rooms? If nothing else, it is doubtful we can label these practices exorcism.

Another interesting case of so-called social exorcism involved George McClain, a social activist in the United Methodist Church and secretary of the Methodist Federation for Social Action. He worked tirelessly against South African apartheid, especially in the Methodist agencies and conferences. He was unsuccessful and came to believe that the institutions themselves might be captive to evil powers. He, with others, conducted a service of exorcism. Subsequently, a key figure in the agency resigned, and policies began to change. Activists became more appreciative of the difficulties faced by the investors in the agency. Perhaps the mutual understanding between the opposing groups was the important step toward positive change. McClain himself does not claim a cause and effect between the exorcism and the positive changes, but references "the logic of the Spirit," which blows where it will.[74]

Tilda Norberg, who cites the above case, even suggests a group exercise in social exorcism, in contrast to a review by the bishop, if an exorcism is warranted. The words suggested to be used are, "Spirit of cynicism, in the name of Jesus we order you to depart from this institution and go to Jesus."[75] However, it seems that a "spirit of cynicism" is a far cry from satanic possession as described in the classic literature on the subject. Similar to our earlier critique of Welker, this broadened definition of demon possession, suggesting the need for exorcism, seems unwarranted and dangerous.

The ministry of deliverance is an authentic part of the liturgical health ministry. But it should be limited to very *rare* situations, which are assessed by mature pastors under strict guidelines. It should never be practiced by solo ministers; it should be in the context of a congregation; and it should not be part of a public healing service.

All these liturgical practices that have been discussed may become resources for a congregation's healing ministry. Understanding their roots and history can form an important part of their rediscovery and use. The sacraments are vehicles of God's transforming power and open us to the Holy Spirit's healing grace. The liturgical rites may be vehicles of God's grace and restoration to wholeness.

5

Educational Programs

Educational health ministries are extremely broad and involve a full range of activities. They are a powerful means through which the church can serve the health needs of its members. Three different constituencies can be served by various approaches: local church members, health care professionals, and the community at large.

CHURCH MEMBER PROGRAMS

Congregational-sponsored education for members includes how to live a healthier lifestyle, change patterns of behavior, make more informed health care decisions, and solve personal problems. Congregations can adopt many creative approaches, such as the following:

- Workshops on personal and professional decision making, divorce recovery, marriage encounter, bioethical quandary issues, stress management, and wellness
- Lectures on patient rights, responsibilities, and informed consent
- Informational materials on health issues and bioethical quandaries
- Shepherding programs by church officers for all church members to keep in touch with ill or homebound persons
- Courses for teenagers on sexuality, family relationships, life goals, marriage, friendship, and pregnancy counseling
- Reading groups on nutrition, meal planning, drug reaction, bioethics, and the spiritual aspects of health care

- Individualized health promotion programs for church members
- Discussion groups for people in transition (job, marital status)
- Health education classes for the general public and church members on such things as stress management, prevention/wellness, spiritual health resources, family life, and bioethical issues
- Visits to research, treatment, and care facilities to become better informed as to what they offer
- Classes by hospital staff on hospital visitation, relationships with attending physicians, and training for volunteer work with persons with disabilities and elderly persons

PROGRAMS FOR HEALTH CARE STUDENTS AND PROFESSIONALS

The second category is education programs for health care professionals, including pastors. The purpose is threefold, namely, to enable all health care professionals to make better use of the full spectrum of health care resources; to better integrate the efforts of the different professionals concerned with health care within a community; and to enable specific professionals, especially pastors, to make better health care decisions. Examples of such programs include the following:

- Symposia on the relation between religion and medicine, church and hospital, pastor and physician.
- Seminars for personnel in hospitals, health care plans, and preventive medicine institutes.
- Consultations on ways that local health care professionals and church members can assist one another.
- Wholistic health care courses, which include theology, medical, nursing, pharmaceutical and social work students, and other related disciplines. These courses would be interdisciplinary, jointly taught and attended by these students. Teachers could be hired part-time or contracted from other institutions. The course work could be complemented by internships for periods of six months to one year for medical students in local churches and for seminary students in primary health care settings. It is important as well to remember continuing education courses for practicing health care professionals; they may discover new, more wholistic health care approaches.
- Courses on the church's role in health and healing, death and dying, aging, bioethics, spirituality and health, addiction, and other related subjects especially for seminarians. For example, as one of

the grant recipients of the PCUSA Health Ministries in Theological Education program, Princeton Theological Seminary sponsored a health awareness week, is currently piloting a new specialized health ministry internship program in cooperation with the Office of Field Education, provides for course electives on health ministry, and collects models of health ministries in the United States and the United Kingdom. An ad hoc committee at the seminary identified five strategic goals for the sustainable development of health ministries at Princeton Seminary: (1) to raise awareness of how preventive health care is necessary in our lives both now and as future pastors, specialized ministers, and educators; (2) to present different kinds of resources for personal and communal health care; (3) to stimulate conversation and foster understanding on the theological importance of health; (4) to demonstrate ways of implementing self-care; and (5) to explore the future steps to ensure a balanced life at seminary by hiring a coordinator of health ministries and the establishment of a wellness center.

As one initiative of the Princeton Seminary Health Ministries Project, the 1998 Festival for Fitness: Healthy Choices, Wholly Living was a weeklong series of events to raise awareness in the entire seminary community about the need for a lifetime of personal care, wholistic health, and physical, psychological, spiritual, and communal wellness. The events included a service of healing, a lunchtime conversation on mental illness, a disability awareness exercise, a festival health fair, a community dinner, a dialogue on healthy relationships, a night of fun and relaxation with a faculty-student basketball game, and CPR training and certification.

- Residential facilities (preferably houses) for ten to fifteen medical, nursing, and theology students, which provide an intentional Christian community for developing understanding and cooperation among these future professionals. These communities could be crucial in changing our understanding of the health care system. Initiatives among students could give rise to research on future health ministries models for cooperation between physicians and clergy, the hospital and the church. (Such a community, Shalom House, was established by National Capital Presbytery Health Ministries in the late 1980s on the grounds of the National Presbyterian Center in Washington, D.C.)

It has been my experience after teaching continuing education courses for health care professionals on integrated health that the place to begin is the preprofessional level. Once patterns of practice and philosophy of a discipline are established, it is difficult to introduce new concepts.

THE CHURCH AS REFERRAL AGENT AND COMMUNITY RESOURCE

The third category of educational programs includes those provided directly by the pastor as well as the use of the church building itself as an educational resource.

By receiving information from resource organizations, local churches can develop resource networks to empower their members to carry forth a health ministry. The church building can be used, for example, as a resource for twelve-step groups or community health inoculation drives. As an institution the church's role can be as subtle as hanging a poster with the phone number of the local battered women's shelter in the women's rest rooms. In this way women who are victims of domestic violence can anonymously seek help. By seeing the poster, they also understand that the church is sympathetic to their plight if they wish to seek counsel and take further action.

Proper referral is a critical role of the church. When a member of the church or the community walks into the pastor's office and reveals that her spouse is an alcoholic and that she is at her wit's end, the pastor can help her get in touch with twelve-step meetings in town, educate her about the recovery process, and arrange an intervention if that seems appropriate. By becoming a member of such resource organizations as the Health Ministries Association, the church not only gains valuable insight into how to expand its own ministry but also positions itself to serve as a resource. Consider how the church pastor could lift the spirits of a demoralized member of the congregation simply by pointing her in the right direction for help.

Church members could volunteer to help the pastor develop a referral network. The right information at the right time can bring healing and empowerment to the body and spirit of God's people. The church can sustain this aspect of health ministry by linking with resource organizations at the denominational, ecumenical, and interfaith levels; and by viewing its very identity as an institution, its own building, pastor, and members as invaluable resources to the wider community.

EDUCATING FOR HEALTH CARE DECISIONS

Returning to the education of local church members, one of the most important ministries is to provide information on controversial issues and training for reaching decisions or positions on health issues. Trying to make decisions in the midst of a crisis about health care options can be disastrous. The church has an important role in helping people make sound decisions. A disciplined method of working through a crisis to a decision is needed. Decisions are not always life threatening but may be life altering. We are not sure who can assist us in making choices. The church can provide workshops led by pastors, health care professionals, social workers, and others to clarify the issues and process for making decisions that affect our lives and those of family members and friends. The educational role of the church becomes even more central as church members try to bring their faith to bear on decisions and perspectives on these knotty and perplexing questions.

Decisions We Face

The number of health care options forces us to make choices. What type of primary health care should we use? Do we join an HMO if our employer gives us a choice, which is less and less the case, or do we use a combination of complementary health care practices and medical care? Do we create our own integrated health care model by using spiritual, medical, and psychological resources that we discover ourselves? What about treatment options? For example, should we have bypass surgery or angioplastic procedures if we have blocked arteries? Or if we are pregnant with a genetically compromised fetus, should we carry the baby to term, put her up for adoption, or have an abortion?

The second area of decision making is the resolution of bioethical dilemmas where decisions involve the use of technological medicine such as in vitro fertilization (IVF) and gene therapy. One of the most important roles of the church is to provide a theological perspective on the procedures being suggested and help people base their decisions on their Christian faith. The church needs to raise the fundamental questions about our headlong pursuit of knowledge unrestrained by ethical and theological considerations.

OPENING PANDORA'S BOX: RESOLVING BIOETHICAL QUANDARIES

Bioethical issues at the edges of life, that is, concerning birthing and dying, especially illustrate the complexity of the options and hard choices. Heretofore, birthing and dying were family events occurring in the home. Now they are medical procedures that involve increasingly complex situations. Pastors are being drawn more and more into a counseling role concerning these issues. The church needs trained people who can lead us through these complicated issues. It is not more spiritual to be ignorant.

Reproductive Technologies

The area of reproductive technologies is especially troubling. There are ten million infertile couples in the United States, many of whom are willing to use any means to fulfill their pursuit of a child including in vitro fertilization, surrogate motherhood, or GIFT (gamete intra-fallopian transfer); for some, even cloning would be considered an option.[1] Furthermore, a growing number of single or lesbian women are freezing their eggs or having IVF in their desire now or in the future to have a child. Each year new techniques are discovered and perfected that give rise to legal battles and ethical dilemmas. The church should not only provide information from knowledgeable experts in the community who lecture on these topics but also offer pastoral counseling and guidance as single people and couples struggle with what technologies are appropriate.

We are fast approaching a point where any and all means of reproducing the human race are accepted. What do we think of technical assistance in procreation? On the one hand, the Roman Catholic position prohibits almost all technical intervention including homologous AID (artificial insemination by donor) (the GIFT procedure is still being debated, but very limited procedures are allowed as an extension of the conjugal act).

The Vatican paper "Instruction on Respect for Human Life in its Origin and on the Dignity of Procreation" expounds on its opposition to IVF and other reproductive interventions. These are seen as undermining maternal love, breaking the conjugal act, and reflecting a basic hostility against life. Curiously, the Roman Catholic Church seems more interested in maintaining the unitive and procreative dimension of intercourse than the exclusivity of one man and one woman. The orthodox Jewish perspective equates AID with adultery. From these religious perspectives, technologies such as surrogate motherhood then become a moot question. Even nonreligious people have a growing concern about our attitudes toward procreation.

Most of the new reproductive technologies separate love, the conjugal act, parenting, and family. Surrogate motherhood, for example, undermines the exclusive nature of one man and one woman. This variation of a ménage à trois brings another woman, if however briefly, into the midst of the intimate experience of a man and a woman, that is, having a child. Tensions will surely develop among these three in all sorts of combinations of jealousy, feelings of inadequacy, that is, not being able to bear a child, or exploitation, that is, bearing one for someone else. It introduces a third person, not only the products of another person but a person in her total-ity. Somehow disembodied elements such as impersonally donated sperm and egg are *less intrusive emotionally* to the unique relationship between one man and one woman.

Many reproductive technologies undermine the role of women. Feminist writers such as Gena Corea have captured one of the problems with the new reproductive technologies: the relegation of women to mother machines.[2] This type of dehumanization is a form of discrimina-tion far harsher than any salary differentials or employment prejudices. In some ways the use of surrogacy instead of adoption may reflect a male hubris for a biological child no matter what emotional cost to the women is involved. It strikes at the core of what it means to be a woman and tears apart her inner self. She is used as an object to satisfy someone else's needs and desires.

Opposition to surrogate motherhood, however, does not equal avoid-ance of all technical assistance in reproduction; in vitro fertilization may be accepted for married couples, but not in other areas. All technical assis-tance for birthing is not immoral nor is it necessary to categorically eliminate all IVF. Its use can be restricted to married couples under very stringent standards as a measure of last resort.

Euthanasia and the Meaning of Death and Dying

Another subject of great concern involves the ethical questions surround-ing the dying process and the end of life. These questions include discontinuing life-support technologies, physician-assisted suicide, and the withdrawal of food and water. These dilemmas should be addressed from the perspective of the meaning of sickness, suffering, death, and dying. Theology deals with ultimate meaning and purpose and can assist us in putting these deep questions of life into perspective. It is not simply under-standing the quandaries but what is behind them that is important.

The underlying issues about euthanasia include the meaning of life, death, and the process of dying whose interpretation affects decisions about forgoing life-extending technologies. Views of life also affect the perspective on euthanasia. These vary from an absolutist perspective (vital-ism)—life is good at any cost with no qualifiers; a prima facie value—life is good but can be laid aside for higher values; or a relative value—life is good only if a certain level of existence is possible.

For some, who is dying makes a difference whether euthanasia is justi-fied. Patients who are in an intensive care unit, marginally alive; are in unremitting pain; are one hundred years old or one day old; have an IQ of

20; or are in other categories of those with diminished autonomy for some are more acceptable or even desirable objects of euthanasia. On the other hand, the twenty-year-old Rhodes Scholar quadriplegic, the mother of four with leukemia, or the stroke patient who is a CEO of a large company may not be considered a prime candidate for euthanasia. Of course, if we take seriously the equality, dignity, and worth of each person as a child of God, these types of distinctions would be unacceptable.

Our view of death per se also influences our acceptance or rejection of euthanasia. If death is a welcome friend who enters as a natural part of life, then euthanasia will be much more acceptable than if we view it as the last enemy to be conquered. If death is the passageway to a better life of immortality rather than the end of all personal existence, then we might even wish to hasten its appearance.

The distinction between the process of dying and the state of death is important in deciding if a treatment is extending a life or prolonging a death. For example, Paul Ramsey, one of the great bioethicists of the twentieth century, refers to the anencephalic (born without a brain) child as already in an irretrievable process of dying, hence justifying no curative treatment. For some people, dying well or choosing how to die may be morally acceptable while choosing death itself may not be.

The question of how death occurs is perhaps the pivotal issue in deciding if a certain death is, in fact, a good death. Within the medical context, death may occur by natural causes; by a person bringing about his or her own death through suicide; or by someone causing another's death against his desire, without his consent, or at his request. It is within this context of how death happens that the morality of euthanasia is considered.

Definitions of Euthanasia

In euthanasia debates, distinctions are usually made between direct/indirect and active/passive euthanasia.[3] Since much controversy surrounds these terms, as Ramsey suggests, it may be impossible to use them any longer in moral analysis.[4] However, it may still be useful to see if there is any meaningful distinction between them and how they shed light on questions about euthanasia, refusal of treatment, and suicide.

Direct euthanasia, bringing about another person's death, can happen in these ways: against his desire; without his consent; or at his request. To understand the moral difference between these acts, we need to distinguish between acts of omission and acts of commission. Omission is the failure to perform a certain act, in this situation not connecting life-support systems or rendering treatment (it is debatable whether supplying food and water is considered treatment, as noted in disagreements about the Cruzan case).[5] Acts of omission are labeled passive euthanasia or letting die. Commission is a positive action, that is, an active intervention to bring about another person's death. Acts of commission here are labeled killing or active euthanasia. (Richard McCormick, a Roman Catholic moral theologian, prefers these two terms to the passive/active distinction.)[6] Hence, bringing about another's death against his desire would be active, involuntary euthanasia. Withdrawal of treatment without a person's consent would be passive, involuntary euthanasia.

Another set of issues thrust into the public debate in the 1990s with the Patient Self-Determination Act centers on refusal of treatment and physician-assisted suicide. It is not only Kevorkian who has been practicing physician-assisted suicide.[7] With advance directives required upon entry into the hospital or nursing home, Christians are looking more and more to their pastors for guidance.

Is suicide wrong in and of itself, or does it depend on the circumstances, that is, the intent and condition of the agent, the consequences, means, and motive? Is it justified or unjustified, rational or irrational? Our answers to some extent are influenced by what we include under the concept of suicide. Bioethicist Tom Beauchamp of Georgetown University suggests that the concept may be so bent out of shape that it is no longer usable. At minimum we should separate it from other related concepts. The primary distinction between euthanasia, refusal of treatment, and suicide is that the latter is solely at one's own hand; it is a direct act, where the primary intent is to end one's physical life.

Refusal of treatment and heroic self-sacrifice should not be included under suicide because this weakens the use of the word. Refusing treatment is choosing the way of dying; committing suicide is choosing death. Put another way, in refusal of treatment the agent is not the primary actor. Refusal of treatment may be an expression of concern on the part of the patient for the health of his or her family. Suicide, on the other hand, is often a hostile, angry act where a person feels that she has lost control of her life. Heroic self-sacrifice is other-regarding, involving a principle or another person. An example is dying while saving a person from a fire or drowning in a lake. What to include under this category is not always clear.

A DECISION-MAKING MODEL

As noted in the discussions about reproductive choices and death and dying, daily decisions are necessary that require examination of one's beliefs and values. The pastor and church educator can assist people in making reasonable and thoughtful decisions that are commensurate with their religious beliefs. The following is a decision-making model that can be used by pastors, hospital chaplains, counselors, and others with their clients and parishioners who face difficult health decisions or can be used directly by the decision maker.

This instrument is designed to assist in reaching sound health care decisions that are consonant with one's values. The goal is to make the best out of tragic situations or complex health decisions. This model outlines the various factors that comprise a decision. It incorporates intuition, emotion, and one's faith perspective, and it acknowledges the mystery and unknown nature of life. It takes into account the fact that not all decisions are clear-cut or made in a linear fashion. The very use of the term "instrument" is misleading, as if one could run through a checklist and arrive at a sound decision. Real life is a lot messier. When belief in God is an important part of our lives, we should be assisted in understanding how our faith can play a practical part in decision making. The pastor and religious counselor have a key role in helping this happen.

Decision making, of course, is not a one-time act but a process. Decisions need to be viewed in relation to their long-term consequences and repercussions, their effect over a lifetime. For example, consider the matter of abortion. An unwed teenager may quickly seek an abortion as an apparent resolution to all her problems but may later suffer guilt and remorse over her decision because of her family upbringing, her values, and her eventual desire to have a child. In assisting people to make decisions, we need to help them think through how they will deal with the ultimate consequences of their decisions.

As we begin to analyze our decisions, we recognize that they have several components: the rational, that is, the facts and information; the emotional, or the feelings; the psychological, which is connected to our mental health and past emotional experiences; and the spiritual/ethical—our values and religious beliefs.

This model is divided into four parts: preparation; analysis; process; and resolution. This is really a description of the stages in decision making.

Preparation

In preparation for decision making, developing one's theology and ethics of health is essential. Ethical sensitivity and morals should be cultivated based on personal, family, community, and national values, which may impact the ultimate decision. Ethical principles such as beneficence and truth telling may clash, necessitating prioritizing of them. However, it is not simply a case of selecting ethical principles but establishing a foundational framework for understanding health, healing, and healers. The religious, spiritual, and transcendent dimensions are important. Here guidance from one's religious denomination and its teachings, relationship with God, and beliefs about God affect the type of decisions made. Prayer and Bible study may put one in touch with the transcendent.

When a pastor first meets with a person facing a decision, she begins by helping the person to be self-aware. Our sexuality influences our self-perception and mode of decision making.[8] Cultural/racial/ethnic origin may influence self-perception and determine the source of one's loyalties and values. One looks, for example, at the contrast between the North American and Latin American understanding of self. For the North American, the task may take precedence over the relationship with other people, while for the Latin American, the opposite is true.

One's sense of self-esteem is also part of preparation for a decision. How much confidence do we have in our own judgments? Do we understand ourselves as unique persons with dignity and worth? Do we recognize our fallibility as we struggle with a decision while maintaining a degree of self-confidence? We must learn to separate who we are from our skills or achievements such as our physical prowess or intellectual gifts in a particular job or position. If we fail to do this, our self-esteem will fluctuate with our performance and hurt our ability to make an autonomous decision.

The third area in preparation is helping people recognize how their life experience equips them to make particular choices; experience produces character, as the apostle Paul stated in Romans 5. Each decision creates a life pattern, which helps us face problems. Hence when the next crisis occurs, we already have experience in making decisions that will contribute to our ability to handle the new situation. The development of moral character as Aristotle suggests results from the practice of certain virtues. Responsibility and accountability are part of this preparation.

Next, in preparing for a particular health decision, gathering information on the various health issues and conditions that affect us is helpful. If, for example, one has colitis, prostate cancer, or arteriosclerosis, gaining information on the physical symptoms and treatments available by reading medical literature, talking to several practitioners, and exploring routine as well as alternative cures leads to a good decision.

The last step in preparation, before the onset of a crisis, is to have a support community in place. Pastors will want to pay particular attention to putting church members in touch with others in the church who have faced similar decisions based on their health conditions; to be sure that they have friends and family surrounding them; and to refer them to any relevant twelve-step groups or community information meetings, seminars, and workshops.

Analysis

Adequate preparation before confronting a problem makes for better choices. When we face an immediate need to make a choice, the first step is to analyze the entire situation. We do this by gathering the data—the medical information about the course of the disease, the symptoms, the prognosis, legal rights, the cost and financial assistance available—and then we assess the wisdom and expertise of the individuals giving us the information.

The second step of analysis is to assess our overall physical condition, how our general health impinges on our decisions. For example, if we have multiple physical problems, we might not risk bypass heart surgery and instead opt for an angioplastic procedure. Determining our primary and secondary health problems is also important in selecting a course of treatment. For example, in treatment decisions about AIDS, often the opportunistic infections—not the AIDS virus itself—demand consideration in treatment plans.

The third step in analyzing a decision is understanding the context of the crisis. For example, deciding to undergo genetic screening for cystic fibrosis can be a very different experience before, rather than during, a pregnancy. As a surrogate decision maker or even for ourselves, we must learn to separate what is a good decision in an abstract sense from what is the right decision in light of the particular circumstances.

As we wrestle with the various choices, we must decide whom we will consult and include in the decision process. We must be aware of how different people interact based on their various areas of expertise. Do we consult our children as well as our spouses about decisions that we are facing? Do we weigh the information from the pastor equally with the doctor's assessment? Do we seek alternative health care practitioners, which raises the previous question of discernment of authentic healing ministries?

Understanding the ethical issues that are part of different decisions is very important. We should distinguish between personal values and objective ethical standards. There is often a gap between theory and practice when choosing ethical principles. One searches how to strike a balance between subjective judgment that any decision is right as long as it is an autonomous one and the perspective that all decisions should be subject to objective standards of right and wrong. One's religious tradition and theology may affect the ranking of particular values. For example, we may cherish both love and truth telling. Do we tell our spouses, whom we love very much, that the doctor says we have six months to live? Or would doing that so adversely affect the relationship that we should not tell our partners? The special relationship of a parent to one's children may create decisions that are prejudicial to one's own health; others' well-being may triumph over personal health. For example, a parent might donate his kidney if it would be a good match for his child.

As we analyze the pros and cons of a particular course of action, projecting the consequences is crucial. Our choices influence the physical course of an illness. These consequences are multiple in nature, involving personal suffering whether it is psychological, physical, or spiritual; vicarious suffering, which may be reproduced in family members or others; and the balance between loss and gain of function or health. For example, if we have a torn cartilage in a knee, we have to weigh the possible future limitations resulting from not having knee surgery against the inherent risk of surgery.

In some situations there is an 80 percent chance of complete recovery, but in 20 percent of the cases death may be the outcome. We may exercise the freedom of autonomy and refuse a treatment in conflict with our value system, knowing that the refusal could shorten our lives. In Roman Catholic theology, the lesser of two evils determines the analysis of tragic choices. The choice is not always black and white between good and evil. For Protestants, choices are not necessarily described as objectively good or bad but rather what is best for all persons in light of tragic choices.

After all this analysis, we should allow for the unexpected, miraculous recovery, for example, from a medically diagnosed terminal illness. If we decide to forgo a life-extending treatment, the faith factor is capricious; we should be open to the God of surprises.

Process

Moving from the analysis of the various dimensions of a decision, we turn to a specific process that can be followed to make the final decision. First, we should use our reason to assess the difference between the right and the good decision. The right decision may be medically correct, but the good decision must be ethically sound. The good decision is a combination of the best medical advice and the honoring of one's highest values. For some people understanding the church's position on a procedure as well as the medical information on the illness is important.

Reason without intuition, however, is sterile. Women often may trust their intuition over and above their reason; intuition is important for all persons. Men call this operating on a hunch. Intuition may also help us get in touch with our conscience. The conscience becomes sharpened through life experience; God can speak to us through it to guide us to the right choice. The conscience may provide the segue to prayer, meditation, and the revelation that comes from a sudden understanding of God's will in a situation.

Reason and intuition should then be joined with our emotions. Some thinkers believe that problems worth solving cannot be done so objectively. This suggests that emotion plays a part in a sound decision. If we agree with thinkers such as Albert Camus, French existentialist (1913–60), our feelings and emotions toward ourselves and others may be the principal factors that sway us.

We do well to recognize that we are not autonomous individuals but part of a community that affects our choices. We should seek the advice of our friends and respected people. We may even seek long-term counseling to assist us in reaching sound decisions. Pastoral counselors should become more versed in helping people clarify their decisions as well as the process used to reach them. They may connect the person with his or her community, whether or not it is religious. For example, people in traditional cultures value consensus from their community very highly and seek it before they proceed with a decision.

The decision process may entail procrastination when we do not feel ready to make an immediate decision. Procrastination may be a temporizing step and is certainly better than total avoidance or denial. In other words, until we feel ready to proceed with a concrete decision, delay may give us the confidence to move ahead. In some cases, rationalization may be used to justify a decision that we know is wrong but we convince ourselves is right because it is the one that we want to choose.

Resolution

The last part of this decision-making model is what we call the resolution or implementation of a decision. Implementing a course of action may be gradual, not in a single step. Once we execute a decision, then we must live with the outcome. Making a decision precludes living with paradox. These paradoxes need to be addressed through conflict resolution where tradeoffs are negotiated. I remember a parishioner at a church I served in New York City who had advanced diabetes and was told if she wanted to live, she had to have her leg amputated. She was paralyzed from reaching a decision because she wanted to both live and *not* have her leg amputated.

The hope is that if the church takes seriously its educational task, then it will equip people to make the best health care decisions. This model is a tool to help people recognize how complex and comprehensive a decision may be.

In summary, educational programs provide a wonderful opportunity for the church to participate in health prevention and wellness and assist people to understand some of the most complicated issues they will ever face. This category of health ministry is foundational for all other areas of health ministry.

6

Support and Advocacy Initiatives

The church's educational programs should be seen as a prerequisite for its involvement in any advocacy initiatives. In other words, the members and clergy should be educated about the issues prior to taking an official stance on such politically divisive issues in bioethics as abortion, physician-assisted suicide, allocation of health care resources, and treatment of special classes of disease. Much of the criticism of Protestant church hierarchies stems from their taking positions on controversial topics. Their stance often comes from a naiveté about the issues. Even when they are knowledgeable, they fail to educate the person in the pew about the reasons for taking a particular position.

Support and advocacy ministries are complementary but interrelated. The key to a particular church's serving as a support community is based on how it functions in a loving, forgiving, and supporting way that affirms the dignity and worth of every member. Concern, support, and the presence of others are very important in the healing process. A person in isolation can languish in loneliness and guilt. The church provides a resource for liberating people from exaggerated individualism and the isolation of contemporary life. The church functions as a community of acceptance and reconciliation. It can testify to the love and healing of God, which are available at all times, not just in moments of crisis. The power of forgiveness, communication, and companionship can often prevent, arrest, and alleviate disease.

As the church fully develops as a loving, forgiving, and accepting community and emerges as a living witness to a theology of wholeness, it is preparing itself for its ministry to persons with special health needs. The church can use many of its traditional functions of Bible study, religious education, prayer, and worship in ministry with these persons. One of the most serious problems faced by ill people is the isolation and loneliness accompanying their problems; there is nothing more restorative than to feel a sense of welcome and acceptance.

Because of its multigenerational nature, the church offers healing in surprising ways, from the laughter of a child to the wise words of an elder. Because of its diversity, the church helps us put our problems in perspective. It can identify with all aspects of the life of a person with special health needs. A very important expression of love is the act of being present with someone in need. This, by itself, can bring enormous healing benefits. However, it may require special training of church members; deep emotions often surface in both the patient and the church member and, if poorly handled, could have a negative effect on both.

The church can express its support in many varied but simple ways. Church members can do cooking, baby-sitting, and shopping; ease the physical discomfort of the patient; and even provide bed-and-breakfast Christian lodging for families of patients hospitalized in nearby institutions. By helping the patient's family, the church reduces some of the anxiety and guilt felt by the patient.

SUPPORT AND ADVOCACY FOR ELDERLY PERSONS—A PRIORITY FOR THE CHURCH

The centerpiece of the church's role in support and advocacy is a ministry with the elderly, one of the largest groups in the church. The church can be involved in several ways. First, with the elderly themselves: valuing and respecting older persons; affirming their accountability as moral agents; and celebrating their gifts. The church can provide accurate information to the elderly about medical facts, especially choices concerning the latest type of treatment and the latest breakthroughs in health care. It can engage in public policy debates about the regulations, guidelines, and laws in the health care arena and work toward the elimination of discrimination based on age. In addition, assistance to those caring for elderly parents and family members in concrete and appropriate ways is crucial. (The Robert Wood Johnson Interfaith Caregivers Program is an effective initiative in this area.)

Most people over age sixty-five think of themselves as the same person they were at forty or fifty, perhaps with diminished physical powers but not ceasing to be oneself. Who willingly describes himself or herself as elderly? The American Association of Retired Persons (AARP) made a brilliant move when it lowered the membership age to fifty, thereby removing the stigma of being old as a criterion for membership. The elderly have contributed to society—its schools, highways, hospitals, churches, and battles to ensure freedom. Now they should receive in their venerable status benefits from society. However, if they become "sick" senior citizens, the United States cannot afford them—its most frequent customers. The irony of modern times is that as we find better and better technologies to sustain and prolong life, we have less regard for the very persons whom our technologies support.

The healing ministry needs to counteract the lack of respect for elderly persons in U.S. culture. From the time of the Social Security Act of 1935, willingness to deal with old age as a problem solidified the perception of old age as just that—a problem. "Retirements and funerals are crude markers for the stark beginning of old age; in between there is a universe of differentiation that remains a cultural wasteland for each to calculate and navigate alone, without the aid of ritual, ceremony, or symbol."[1] In 1998 there were 25 million people over age sixty-five in the United States, representing 11 percent of the population. By the year 2030, an estimated 21 percent of the U.S. population will be over sixty-five. Moreover, we have divided that group by labels: sixty-five to seventy-four years are the elderly; seventy-five to eighty-four years are the aged; and eighty-five and over the very old. The implication of this categorization is that if you are part of the last group, you are beyond the pale. This is not only the case in the United States. For example, the National Health Service in Britain uses age as a sufficient criterion to exclude certain persons from such medical care as kidney dialysis. We should note, however, there are some dramatic changes taking place with the elimination of mandatory retirement at age sixty-five and the use of retirees as consultants.

Valuing and Respecting the Elderly

The question often asked is, Why were the elderly accorded respect in the past and still are in some societies? One possible answer is the presence or absence of writing technologies. In literate societies, books, computers, and microfilm replace human memory, although some literate societies still hold the aged in esteem. For example, older Kalahari Kung women are treated with respect because others look to them for the stories of the past, whether mythic or historical. They know the histories and scandals of people living and dead and the folk tales kept alive by word of mouth from one generation to the next. Older people have specific contributions: "Long after their productive years have passed, the old people are fed and cared for by their children and grandchildren. The blind, the senile, and the crippled are respected for the special ritual and technical skills they possess."[2]

A second factor is that mechanized technologies are replacing craftspersons' skills, so compulsory retirement is a way of substituting machines for people. Devaluing the elderly may result from new workplace relations and sheer physical endurance to keep the economic machine humming. New technologies such as computers tend to make obsolete previously valued skills.

In addition, the elderly are devalued because worth has been tied to physical prowess and mental capabilities. From a religious faith perspective, valuing and involving people at all stages of life are necessary. Carl Jung expressed it, "The afternoon of life must also have significance of its own and cannot be merely a pitiful appendage to life's morning."

The biblical perspective on aging and the elderly is very positive. Although Jesus said that we must become as little children in order to enter the realm of heaven, the comment was connected not with chronological age but with a faith and openness to the future and new realities. This youthful attitude is possible at any time of life. Unfortunately, despite the strong biblical and theological reasons for revering the elderly,[3] religious communities have not always responded adequately to the needs of the elderly (who represent 50 percent of the membership in churches and synagogues—more than twice their percentage in the general population) or used their gifts and experiences to the fullest extent possible. There is a tremendous lack of religious education and materials for adults over sixty-five years. Of more than two hundred accredited theological institutions in the United States and Canada, only a half dozen have full-time faculty persons in the area of religion and aging.[4] Silent disapproval (even in religious communities that think it fit to lift up in prayer any and every human reality) most often accompanies the real diminishments that happen by physical decline, by failure in productivity, by living longer than one's generation, or even simply by looking old. Scripture and the teaching of religious traditions that value the elderly can change society's perceptions.

Valuing older persons is a way of supporting them. This valuing is grounded in enhancing the dignity and worth of every person as a child of God. Respect for persons is independent of abilities, intellect, physical strength, or beauty; the internal rather than the external person. This valuing applies to all but especially the comatose or frail elderly. There is a danger, however, with the frail to deny the reality of frustration and inhibition that may result from weakening physical powers.

It is important to admit that as we age, we all feel a certain sense of loss. In the field of rehabilitation medicine an acknowledgment of the loss of particular functions through accident or disease is compared to death and referred to as body loss and bereavement. This perspective is instructive in understanding some of the effects of the aging process. How we deal with the grief and sense of loss for the parent we knew, who has become the child we once were, may affect how we respond to our own aging.

The Elderly as Full Moral Agents

Affirming the elderly as responsible moral agents can serve as a corrective for society's general paternalistic approach. The expressions we hear for old age such as "years of fulfillment," "sunset years," and "the winter season" are in contrast to much of our understanding of God's calling. Karl Barth wrote, "He is always at one point in his life process which even at its end is still a 'becoming' even though at its very beginning it is already a 'perishing.' God's claim on us is now as though it were the first and last."[5] God confronts us continually, not just in youth but old age, so we are constantly called in responsibility to step out of the past into freedom.

The apostle Paul captured this view when he wrote, "Forgetting what lies behind and straining forward to what lies ahead, I press on toward the goal for the prize of the heavenly call of God in Christ Jesus" (Phil. 3:13–14). That was written in the spirit of youthful verve despite the fact that Paul wrote the letter to the Philippians in prison when he was old. As we grow older, reminiscing and inactivity may project that we are like ones already dead. But, as Barth says, as we recognize the proximity of the coming Judge, it becomes even more important to act. "Now God said to Abram, 'Go from your country and your kindred and your father's house to the land that I will show you'" (Gen. 12:1). By that departure, he became the father of believers. In the psalms, for example, the prayer of an old man is of one who still looks to proclaim God's power.[6]

Probably one of the most important areas for moral agency of the elderly concerns decisions related to death and dying. Part of our own fear of aging, as well as our eschewing those who are older, is our fear of death—the loss of hope and the existence of a future. The church can proclaim our hope in eternal life, which may do more than anything else to empower elderly persons. Many religious traditions emphasize the resurrection and fulfillment of life after death with the promise of a continuation of life in a fuller and richer way. The doctrine of the resurrection and eternal life in Christian theology, as Thomas Aquinas described it, connotes that the past, present, and future are always the present in God's time, that is, now. Time is a continuum stretching into eternity. This understanding may alter how we feel about the so-called sunset or last years; they become as a prelude to entering into life in its fullness, not a discontinuity. Despite a belief in eternal life, death is the last enemy to be conquered. People should be allowed to decide how they want to die.

Affirming the Gifts of Elderly Persons

A strength of the church is its possibility of using the many gifts of each person for enriching the human community. The elderly generally have the two gifts of time and experience—time to be with others, time to talk, time to reflect, time to understand, time to appreciate, time to develop relationships of depth and meaning.

In contemporary Western society, time is a precious commodity, with very few willing to share it. The busyness that marks our lives, which produces high levels of stress, is a result of overprogramming in a frantic search for meaning. By virtue of retirement and a general acceptance that people over age sixty-five need no longer work at full-time positions, time may be their gift to share with others.

The elderly may also be able to share experience and wisdom. Wisdom does not automatically come with passing years. It is something that must be gained through perspective and reflection on life's events and facts. Not all of us learn from our past mistakes; we may keep repeating them. The passage of years does not automatically produce wisdom, but experience often accompanies it. In Romans 5, Paul referred to suffering and tribulation as producing endurance, endurance bringing forth patience, patience developing character, which in turn produces hope. Experience in one sense teaches us that we can endure, no matter what the crises or circumstances. The elderly can share those insights with us as the church learns more effective ways to incorporate their gifts.

Assisting the Caregivers of Aging Parents

The concrete support and assistance by church members to caregivers of aging parents offer a lifeline. The assistance is not only providing respite care from their duties but also helping caregivers clarify expectations. When decisions are made about caring, it is important at the outset to define boundaries of care. Doing this may appear to conflict with the Christian perspective on covenant relationships, but without boundaries, burnout and resentment may occur. It is startling to realize that one in four workers provides care for aging relatives, averaging twelve to thirty-five hours per week. In 1994, 12 million persons sixty-five and over were limited by chronic conditions necessitating the assistance of caregivers,[7] forming the picture of the "sandwich generation," middle-age workers who are sandwiched between their children and their parents. Resentment and guilt are common responses to the burden of caring for elderly parents, whose aging somehow threatens our own sense of mortality; "respect" is not a word we frequently use.

Caring for our elders throws into bold relief past family dynamics and often exacerbates any dysfunction. Edwin Friedman, rabbi and family therapist, points out that early family patterns of relating become intensified when the parent becomes the child: "Parents who tended to infantilize their children as they raised them are likely to receive a similar approach in return from their children who now must parent them."[8] The point is that by breaking that cycle and creatively changing the relationships, one's own children may benefit.

The church may assist people in making hard decisions about the care of elderly parents. Where possible when faced with competing needs, first honor the needs that will not violate the needs of others. A rule of thumb is that the most vulnerable are those who deserve the greatest care. However, if providing such care will cause an undue burden, that may be a justifying criterion for deciding not to care for an ill parent in one's home. The consequences of an aged parent living in the home must be weighed so that the whole family system is not disrupted as a result. The tragic destruction of a family by the wrong decisions about the care of ill parents may be avoided if different ways of meeting needs are considered. Alternatives should take into account immediate as well as long-term effects on a family. A husband opposed to his mother-in-law's living in his house, for example, might lead to divorce in the family if she lived there. In that instance, a parent can live in a nursing home, but the adult child can visit the parent daily as a way of offsetting the deepest fear of nursing home existence—that of being abandoned.

JUSTICE-BASED HEALTH CARE REFORM

Another crucial area of advocacy is justice-based health care reform. Given the failure of systematic health care reform, it is urgent for the sake of the 44 million uninsured and the others lacking medical services that the church speak out against these injustices.[9] Most major denominations have developed moral foundations for systemic health care reform. In 1994 the Interreligious Health Care Access Group launched a health care reform campaign based on ethical principles. Health care is a justice issue here and around the world as to how we allocate our health care resources. The church is called to perform a prophetic role in helping to assure that all needy persons receive a fair minimum standard of health care. The inclusion of all people is itself a form of advocacy, but changing laws, working on universal health care coverage, and lobbying for the marginalized are part of the church's mission in health care.

By applying the philosophical concepts of justice, one can begin to construct a health care system that accounts for the needs of all people. A call to justice without its implementation is hollow. Justice as fairness and comparative and compensatory justice are appropriately applied to the health care arena. If we apply the principle of comparative justice, a decent fair minimum standard of health care needs to be established for a particular community so that all members of the community receive that level of health care. This is not an absolute worldwide standard, but a standard relative to a particular geographic area. For example, a CAT scan in every community may not be a necessity. However, safe drinking water, adequate food and housing, inoculations, prenatal services, curative drugs, and annual physical examinations would be included under a decent fair minimum of health services.

On the other hand, compensatory justice demands that people who are at risk or ill due to genetic, socioeconomic, gender, age, or race factors merit a larger percentage of the total health care resources by virtue of their greater need and vulnerability. Weak, powerless, and marginalized persons need a larger share of the health care resources to offset their disadvantages; our neighbor in need as pictured in the good Samaritan parable.

A Sample of Denominational Perspectives on Health Care Reform

Many Christian churches have developed positions that reflect a justice-based health care reform platform. The key question is, How can we engage local pastors and members in the debate about fair allocation of health care resources? There are excellent denominational materials on this subject, but the person in the pew rarely sees them. These materials emphasize wholistic health care and the need for universal access to quality health care, regardless of race, gender, or economic status. What is missing in almost all these statements is implementing strategies, which take into account the political and power dynamics that prevent an inclusive health care system. However, the church's involvement in health care reform highlights the importance of advocacy as part of a health ministry.

The Health Care Access Campaign. Thirty-two faith groups launched the Interreligious Health Care Access Campaign to promote systemic reform of the U.S. health care system. However, there is not uniformity in all issues among the participating groups. For example, following the Lutherans' "emphasis of the importance of individual conscience over institutional authority,"[10] the Evangelical Lutheran Church of America (ELCA) asked members to consider the campaign's working principles, compare them with proposals from the president and Congress, and then ask for God's guidance in one's deliberations, acting in Christian love toward one another.[11]

The Health Care Access Campaign focused on a national health care system that would do the following:

- Serve everyone living in the United States, guaranteeing all people access to care in the nation.
- Provide the whole U.S. population comprehensive benefits, including prevention services and health promotion; primary and acute care; extended care and rehabilitation; and mental health care.
- Set a prospective budget for payments to health care institutions from federal funds, drawing financial support from the broadest possible resource base, in a way that assures services for all parts of a region. However, this does not imply a "nationalized" medical service or ending administrative control by independent health care providers.
- Set a national budget for health education and wellness promotion.
- Provide quality service and payment processes based on principles of equity and efficiency.
- Consider the compensation, retraining, and placement of health care workers displaced by changes within the system due to reform.
- Reduce the burden of malpractice litigation.
- Curb significantly the current rapid inflation in the cost of providing medical services; but where possible, assure the freedom of consumers to choose medical providers.
- Provide federal leadership in health promotion by assessing the health impact of standard of living issues such as housing, nutrition, physical fitness, environmental safety, and sanitation.
- Promote effective and safe innovation and research in medical techniques, research on the delivery of health services, and on the health practices of individuals and families.[12]

This challenging set of goals, which none could fault, appears disconnected from reality because some aims are mutually exclusive; freedom to choose health plans and reduction of costs in the current climate are not possible.

Presbyterian Church (U.S.A.). Although the Health Care Access Campaign represented a broad set of aims, denominations such as the Presbyterians were concerned that health care reform should be grounded in a broad definition of health as a value. From their perspective, good health includes physical, mental, and spiritual well-being. It is both a gift of God and a social good of special moral importance. Its value derives from the Hebrew and Christian Scriptures. Good health is viewed as a basic need and an essential purpose of human and societal development, which allows us to fulfill our role in society. We have personal responsibility for our health. This perspective is grounded in our moral obligation—our private and public duty—to value and care for our own and others' health. We are stewards of God's creation and need to adopt healthier lifestyles. In addition, society as a whole and its constituent public, private, and voluntary organizations have a moral obligation to promote a healthy environment and to ensure the availability of health-giving resources for everyone. The free-market system is insufficient to provide the adequate supply and equitable distribution of these resources. We are responsible to work toward the best achievable standards and the most effective performance of the health care system.

The Presbyterians, along with others, embraced the principles of a National Medical Plan that would include eligibility, benefits, financing, reimbursement, resource development and delivery system structure, policy and administration, assessment and assurance of quality, management of use, cost containment, choice, linkages, and a transition plan from the old to the new system.

American Baptist Church. The Baptists adopted a resolution concerning the current health care crisis. The General Board of the American Baptist Churches' "Resolution on Health Care for All" elaborated on its 1975 "Policy Statement on Health Care." In this statement, parallel to other denominations, health care was viewed as a right, not a privilege, with the goal of universal access to comprehensive benefits.[13] The American Baptists propose a Christian model that involves "health, healing and wholeness, and defines health as the state of a person in Christ, a new creature made whole by spiritual conversion."[14] A Christian model leads us to a different understanding of health; it is not a perfect state of being. Health as wholeness involves the acceptance of the limitations of being a finite creature in a divinely created but fallen order. For the Baptists and others, the crisis in the U.S. health care system is a result of the current "patchwork system" of health care providers, health office workers, health support staff, insurers, and payers who function uncoordinated. The resolution further states that the crisis is economic since the United States pays more for health care than many other industrialized nations and receives less for its money. Efforts at shifting costs among government agencies, private insurers, and individual payers have created enormous additional bureaucratic and regulatory costs beyond the costs for health care itself without bringing the 44 million uninsured into a plan.

United Methodist Church. The United Methodist Church (UMC) echoes the need for a radical overhaul of the health care system in the United States. It calls for legislation that will provide universal access to quality health care while controlling costs.[15] It believes that its mission is to continue the redemptive ministry of Christ's healing—a wholistic ministry of spiritual, mental, emotional, and physical healing.

The UMC contends that the "excesses" of the present medical system have started to erode many of the technological achievements that have cured severe illness and prolonged life. The poor, the aging, women, children, persons with disabilities, and persons of color are most at risk in this system as the report substantiates by verifying statistics on the health indices of marginalized groups. Even the middle class has difficulty finding affordable, quality care when catastrophic illness hits. As the church report points out, not only consumers but other segments of society are unhappy—corporations, unions, doctors, and hospitals.

As an advocate, the UMC has worked with the Interreligious Health Care Access Campaign previously mentioned. It affirms the role of Christlike care in institutions that provide direct health services by units of the UMC as well as the development of a curriculum on universal health care advocacy suitable for its seminaries. In addition, it resolved in 1984 to join with the international community, represented by the World Health Organization, in affirming health for all by the year 2000 as one of the most important social goals of the twentieth century.[16]

Episcopal Church, U.S. Not all denominations jumped on the universal access and Health Care Access Campaign. Contrary to an optimistic stance favored by other denominations, which offer the church as the knight in shining armor to a nation in distress, the Episcopal Commission with surprising deprecation asserted that the church cannot solve the health care problems confronting this nation. Despite its demurral that the church cannot offer a cure, the commission called upon each diocese to address the health care crisis in an aggressive way by articulating a moral position. The church "can and must be responsible for health promotion and disease prevention."[17]

Like other denominations, the Episcopal Church supports a wholistic approach to health. It opposes biomedicine's separation of body and spirit, which views the body as a machine that can be analyzed in terms of "the functioning of the different body parts down to the molecular level."[18]

The Episcopal Church's Commission on Health's 1994 report refrained from making a comprehensive statement about health care reform because "even the most careful work might be outdated" given the turbulent state of affairs in health care. The Episcopal Church opted instead to couch its position in a five-point theological statement that would "begin a conversation" about health care within the church, highlighting such issues as domestic violence, prolongation of life, health care for women, including reproductive health and menopause, and clergy wellness.

The seventy-first General Convention of the Episcopal Church in 1994 adopted five principles as the church's position on health care. The first four principles mirror other mainline denominations' positions. The first principle promotes "universal access to quality, cost effective, health care services" for everyone, even for those "requiring long term care." The second principle, "quality health care," is defined to include programs in preventive medicine, "where wellness is the first priority." The third principle stipulates that "quality health care" includes interdisciplinary and interprofessional components to insure the care of the whole person—physiological, spiritual, psychological, and social. Balanced distribution of health care resources "so that no region of the country is underserved" informs the fourth principle.

The fifth principle sets it apart from other denominations. It allows the hastening of death in the case of the incurably ill person who is in acute pain and distress. Medication to alleviate the pain should not be denied on the grounds that death might come sooner. Therefore, the guideline is clear that medication is to be given not to end the person's life but to bring comfort and some quality of life even if that brings death sooner.[19] (How much quicker and by what means are precisely the questions addressed by the 1997 Supreme Court ruling, outlawing physician-assisted suicide but giving states a great deal of leeway.) It supports its position theologically on the grounds that "followers of the crucified and risen Christ do not place the highest value on mere biological existence."[20]

It views its position on health care or health care reform not as definitive but as a "work in progress," the beginning of a conversation drawing in Episcopal ethicists, liturgists, theologians, physicians, nurses, research scientists, and health care workers of all kinds "so that voices from every corner of our communion may be heard and heeded." The purpose is to engage the church over time in serious discourse about Christian social responsibility in the area of health care.

Roman Catholic Church. Perhaps as a result of its centralized authority and size, in contrast to most Protestant denominations, the Roman Catholic Church offers one of the most comprehensive positions on health care reform. Its sweeping statement, "Comprehensive Health Care Reform: Protecting Human Life, Promoting Human Dignity, Pursuing the Common Good," was issued in a 1993 Resolution of the Catholic Bishops of the United States.

The Catholic Health Association assembled a detailed proposal for "Systemic Healthcare Reform," which concludes that health care reform is essentially a debate about values.[21] The Catholic Health Association embodies six values in its reform proposal, which are summarized here:

1. *Health care is a service.* It is more than a business and is an essential social good, a service to persons in need. Health is not "a commodity exchanged for profit." (This statement falls short of the Presbyterians' position that health is a fundamental good, not simply an instrumental one.)

2. *Every person is the subject of human dignity.* Universality of access means that all Americans have a right to health care. "The importance of health care to human dignity insists that all people have a right to basic and comprehensive health care."

3. *Public policy must serve the common good.* We cannot be interested only in the rights of a few, but we must be committed to the best interests of our nation and communities. Service to the common good was basic to the United States and forms an important part of biblical and other national traditions that must be recovered. "Rediscovery of the common good is critical to the future of health care as well as to all our social systems."

4. *The needs of the poor have a special priority.* "The wealthy and the well should care for the poor and the sick. Since programs for the poor too often become poor programs, a reformed health care system should tie the fate of the poor to that of all Americans."

5. *There must be responsible stewardship of resources.* Stewardship is an individual requirement so that health care reform "requires the introduction of economic discipline into the health care delivery system. Overall spending must be within realistic political limits."

6. *Tasks should be performed at appropriate levels of organization.* All levels of government should be involved with federal authority creating a national health care community; response to local diversity

should be through state involvement so that a range of choice is protected and a variety of plans assured.

The Catholic Health Association focuses on "delivery reform" as one of the first steps to health care reform. The current delivery system "is deficient primarily because it is fragmented, costly and often restricted." Financial incentives are structured to discourage providers from cooperation, and there is little integration among primary care, acute care, and long-term care settings. Health promotion and preventive care are often not covered. The current system lacks internal economic discipline, forcing purchasers to use costly and demoralizing external controls on physicians and health care facilities. Reform proposals will succeed only in concert with a reformed delivery system.

At the heart of the Catholic proposal is the Integrated Delivery Network (IDN), a set of providers organized to deliver a coordinated continuum of health care services including health promotion, preventive care, home care, hospice and rehab, hospital care, specialty care, and primary care. This well-conceived plan recommends that IDNs would operate under either contractual or ownership arrangements by several IDNs, which compete for enrollees on the basis of quality and service. They would be managed by a variety of entities, including hospitals, physicians, former insurance companies, or combinations of these groups. IDNs would be organized to take financial risk for providing a comprehensive benefit package to an enrolled population. The IDN would receive risk-adjusted capitalized payments based on the demographic and epidemiological characteristics of the IDN's enrolled population. It would be held accountable for improving or maintaining the health status of its enrolled population.

These IDNs would receive their risk-adjusted capitated payments from an independent, politically insulated State Health Organization (SHO). The SHO would charter and monitor the IDNs and be responsible for ensuring that each IDN delivers the scope and quality of services guaranteed under the law. It does not, however, dictate the IDNs' contractual arrangements or methods of payment with providers.

An independent, politically insulated National Health Board (NHB) would ensure overall order in the system and would define a comprehensive benefit package and establish a national health care budget. The NHB would receive funds from a dedicated national health care trust fund to pay for the system and, in turn, send those funds to the SHO on the basis of risk-adjusted capitation payments for the covered population.

The rest of the Catholic proposal addresses the issue of cost to the consumer and eventually to the nation as a whole. It outlines a rather elaborate cost savings plan and concludes by stating, "The proposal will save the U.S. economy large amounts of money annually. If the reformed system reduces the rate of spending by only two percent each year, a total of $856 billion will be saved by the end of eight years."[22]

The hope is that these positions of various denominations will encourage reflection on the importance of church involvement in reforming health care in this country so that *all* people may be included in the U.S. health care system, certainly the most important moral issue facing us today. By examining two very different, but related issues of justice and concern, that is, the needs of the elderly and those excluded from adequate health care, we strike at the heart of Christ's preferential option for the poor and the call to the church to be a voice for the voiceless.

7

The Church Delivers
Wholistic Health Care

S everal types of direct health services can form part of the church's
health ministry: (1) medical mission hospitals and clinics;[1] (2) primary
health care in a wholistic or integrated mode; (3) behavioral and mental
health care through counseling and spiritual analysis for inner healing; and
(4) prevention of illness, especially of addiction in all its forms through
varied approaches. The church can help in providing health care, especially
in light of the shrinking pool of caregivers.[2] One illustration is the
National Federation of Interfaith Volunteer Caregivers program. In this
program, the church trains volunteers to provide support services that
enable ill or elderly persons to remain at home. Why should the church
abandon health care to the major managed health care corporations? It
should become a key player in prevention and meeting long-term health
needs, not simply be the ambulance picking up the dead and wounded. It
can assist people so that they can die at home, if they wish, instead of
in hospitals and institutions.[3] This chapter, rather than discussing the
more traditional health care services, focuses on new models of health care
delivery as well as the church's unique ministry in the area of mental health
and prevention.

THE CHURCH REDEFINES PRIMARY HEALTH CARE

The definition of health influences what is included under primary health
care. The Christian Medical Commission of the World Council of
Churches defined health as "a dynamic state of well-being of the individual and of the society; of physical, mental, spiritual, economic, political

and social well-being, in harmony with each other, with the material environment and with God."[4] It defined primary health care as "a system in which people take part in defining their own needs and setting their own priorities for meeting these needs which have to do with health in its broadest sense."[5] Health care should be community based, starting with meeting people's needs. A ministry of healing is an act of obedience through which the church becomes a community of concern responding to needs within its midst. The church has three main avenues of healing given to it by God—medicine, counseling, and prayer. To fail to exercise its stewardship of these resources is to neglect the will of God.[6] The commission agreed that the church is called to be more than a gathering place for worship and goodwill; it must include activities of sharing and caring for one another and the community of which it is a part.[7]

The pioneering work of Dr. Granger Westberg in the 1960s and 1970s in the United States to establish whole-person care clinics in churches set the agenda for how churches could reach out beyond their doors with health-giving resources in primary care. Four to six centers were established in the greater Chicago area and underwritten by a Kellogg Foundation grant. Emphasizing preventive health programs, patient education seminars, and a comprehensive team, Westberg was the catalyst for dozens of church-based health care enterprises.

A typical example of wholistic health care was the Capitol Hill Wholistic Health Center, which existed from 1982 to 1993 in the Lutheran Church of the Reformation in Washington, D.C. It principally served church members and people who worked on the Hill, almost entirely a middle-class clientele. The center's purpose was spelled out in its founding statement: "Total health of people is a function of the interrelationship between mind, body, and spirit; that moral, ethical and faith-related decisions are inseparably connected to a proper approach to health; that lifestyle, environment, and behavior patterns influence the total health of the individual, hence wholistic healthcare should be delivered."[8]

The Center offered personal counseling and health education to help the patient become responsible for getting and staying well. The staff consisted of a board-certified family physician, a pastoral counselor, and a nurse practitioner, who provided traditional, acute, and chronic medical care. A nonprofit organization, the Center relied on patient fees to meet expenses for its broadly defined primary care services including both conventional and "creative" medical care; clinical testing and treatment; individual, marriage, and family counseling; nursing services, which included health assessment and teaching; a Health Planning Conference in which patient, doctor, counselor, and nurse formed a team to develop a personal treatment plan for wellness in body, mind, and spirit; seminars in stress management, nutrition, disease prevention, family life, and disciplines teaching personal responsibility for health care and addiction prevention and treatment.[9] The director, Bryon Mayberry, served on the National Capital Presbytery Health Ministries board in the 1980s when I was its director. I knew firsthand the struggles they encountered about attracting patients and securing funding. The third-party payment system in the United States is not structured to cover these types of services.

INNER HEALING

These more wholistic health care systems are very important, yet the church has some unique contributions in the area of mental health. In the U.S. context this is generally translated into pastoral counseling, but in some circles this is referred to as inner healing, which some believe is a necessary prelude to physical healing.

Although the church's perspective on primary health care is wholistic, different facets of health care need to be examined. Healing, as stated, is a movement toward wholeness. To bring about wholeness, inner healing is necessary, which includes the need for forgiveness and reconciliation in broken relationships. Inner healing is wholistic in approach and understands people as a unity of body, mind, and spirit.[10] Inner healing means healing of the intellectual, volitional, and affective makeup of a person—healing past memories and emotional hurts. For example, concealed anger may kill the spirit and hurt the body. A purely medical approach to illness, whether through drugs or surgery, that does not address the underlying causes of the illness has limited effectiveness. Inner healing may be needed before a physical cure can take place. Healing may mean comforting and supporting persons experiencing an incurable disease. Even though cure is not possible, an inner peace and acceptance may result from the presence and love of others.

Healing as Mending Relationships

An effective way of inner healing is a process called faith imagination in which we invite Jesus Christ to join us in the place where we hurt. For example, we may return to a painful childhood scene and imagine Jesus holding us. Jesus may enter into our deepest pain, and there Christ's love may transform, forgive, and redeem us. The mending of relationships may involve the healing of painful memories, or the transforming of anger and resentment by peace and joy. This truth is especially evident for the recovery of sexual abuse and incest victims and persons suffering from traumatic stress syndrome. Their painful, often suppressed memories may inhibit their ability to be healed unless they face, accept, and eventually overcome their trauma.

Faith imagination is linked to imaging in general, which has often been used effectively for pain control. A hospital chaplain I met years ago at the Veterans Administration Hospital in Washington, D.C., ran a control experiment using imaging as a way of pain control in cancer patients vis-à-vis medication used by the medical staff. The patients who practiced imaging were more pain-free. His study opened up the medical staff to accept new techniques.

Part of inner healing is the restoration of relationships in which God uses one person to help another feel whole. Denis Duncan, a British pastoral theologian, gives an interesting illustration of the right kind of healing relationship by using the story of Jesus' encounter with Zacchaeus.[11] Jesus first invited Zacchaeus to come down from the tree so that they could engage on the same level. A healing relationship is built as one moves toward another. However, the person needs his or her own space to reveal the inner self, which should be protected by confidentiality. In the case of Jesus, we do not really know what was said in his conversation with Zacchaeus, but we know that Jesus established immediate and direct communication with him.

We must start where the persons are without judgment about why they got themselves into a particular problem. Healing relationships involve sympathy and empathy. "Being with" is at the heart of what Jesus had to offer Zacchaeus; while others were judging whether Jesus had any business being with a tax collector, Jesus was ministering to Zacchaeus's real needs. This seizing of the moment that Duncan describes is reminiscent of the description by Donald Capps, pastoral theologian at Princeton Theological Seminary, of the pastoral care performed by most parish pastors, acts that "involve brief, time-compressed encounters . . . in the context of a life crisis."[12]

Forgiveness Is Key to Inner Healing

Restoring relationships, which is necessary for inner healing, is linked to forgiveness. The results of forgiveness are reconciliation and freedom, which are health giving. Reconciliation is connected with loving our enemies. Forgiveness shows that the world is destined to move not toward greater disorder and darkness but toward redemption. Human beings can respond to inhuman acts by being sane and civilized—forbearing. Reconciliation begins between individuals, then impacts systems. God's forgiveness enables us to forgive others. Forgiveness is not some interesting sidelight of the Christian life but is at the heart of what it means to be a Christian. However, forgiveness is a work as well as a grace.

Often our inability to accept forgiveness is rooted in the self: self-abasement, self-abhorrence, self-accusation, self-defeat, self-disparagement, self-hatred, self-pity, and self-torture are fertile ground for the unforgiving spirit. Accepting God's forgiveness can transform hatred of self. God's incomprehensible love and salvation are at the heart of the church's message of health.[13]

We can forgive ourselves for the wrong we do as we accept God's forgiveness as a sign of grace in the face of repeated failure in thought, word, and deed. Being forgiven and forgiving others are health giving; we move toward wholeness. We are set free to put the past behind—to put aside hate and judgmental attitudes that eat away inside us and replace them with compassion and understanding that heal the inner spirit.

Therapeutic Counseling and Spiritual Healing

As mentioned earlier, inner healing includes the healing of memories. This introduces the question of the interface between therapeutic counseling and spiritual healing since both deal with the inner life. First, all the wisdom and insight from psychology and psychiatry should form a part of a healing ministry (even if not overtly Christian). A split between the tools and skills of psychiatry and the resources of religious practices should be avoided. In addition to the clinical dimension of counseling, the pastoral aspect recognizes the spiritual component of the counselor-client relationship. This emphasis is important in terms of placing the healing ministry in the center of pastoral theology; in the past it has too often been subsumed under the clinical. Counseling as part of a healing ministry recognizes the work of the Holy Spirit at the center of the counseling relationship. However, professional training before offering counseling services is vital because the potential abuses from ignorance are many.[14]

Pastoral counseling should be a natural bridge between medicine and theology. Yet that has not always been the case. Under Seward Hiltner, pastoral counseling was centered in the Clinical Pastoral Education (CPE) model, which was hospital- rather than parish-based. CPE places a group of seminarians in a hospital setting to understand themselves in relation to others, provide pastoral care to patients, and work under the supervision of a certified CPE chaplain. It is most frequently centered on death and dying issues in a crisis setting rather than dealing with broad health care issues.

Leaders such as George Fitzgerald, using parish-based CPE, are helping change the medical model emphasis. The CPE model needs to be reenergized to take into account the new insights concerning the centrality of spiritual resources for healing. In addition, the crucial, multifaceted role of the chaplain as a member of the hospital healing team needs to be recognized and legitimized within the clinical setting. Hospital chaplains have performed effectively numerous roles, and the church owes a debt of gratitude to their outstanding work. In the 1980s and 1990s hospital chaplains were viewed more and more as ethicists or liaison with different constituencies within the medical setting rather than pastoral caregivers. In fact, most CPE students are strictly instructed not to pray with the patients or even initiate religious conversations. This is not to suggest that chaplains are to be evangelists or, worse yet, proselytizers, but surely there is some middle ground. Now at the initiative of the hospital, the interface of spirituality and health has returned as part of their portfolio, and more and more chaplains are responding to this situation.[15]

A discussion of pastoral counseling and theology is beyond the purview of this book. Yet one should note the dramatic shifts in the field since Hiltner's day. Theology, on the one hand, is being reintroduced into the field by such scholars as Deborah van Deusen Hunsinger at Princeton Theological Seminary; she has brought together such seemingly disparate thinkers as C. G. Jung and Karl Barth, who though both in Switzerland seemed to have little to say to each other. Her paradigm is based on God's otherness while respecting the experience of the human psyche. Her plea for pastoral counseling to become interdisciplinary is an important one,[16] which would benefit as well from the inclusion of ethics and spirituality as part of the mix. Certainly pastoral care could be enriched by the breadth of theology by grounding the discipline in more than pop psychology. The distinctions between sinner and victim are important and also surface in the contrast between the charismatic's language of inner healing and the counselor's vocabulary of therapy and self-discovery.[17] One of the primary questions being raised concerns the goal of counseling. Is it a right relationship to God or to self? Are the two compatible? Learning to love oneself appears to be at the heart of Christ's twofold command, but the way of self-knowledge is believed to be through loving God, not only through being introspective.

The Clinical Theology Movement
Combines Counseling and Spiritual Healing

In the United Kingdom the work of Frank Lake in the late 1950s and 1960s broke new ground with his clinical theology that combined

Christian theology with modern psychiatry. In other words, he joined counseling and spiritual healing and brought together pastoral care and spiritual healing. Lake founded and directed the Clinical Theology Association, which is still controversial among pastoral theologians in Britain.[18] Some ministers have difficulty seeing counseling as a form of healing ministry because of their reaction to Lake's evangelical stance.[19] His landmark book *Clinical Theology* (1966) was based on perspectives gained from groups of clergy and doctors meeting in dioceses for seminars in human relations, pastoral care, and counseling. Their purpose was to determine how pastors could become more effective pastoral counselors.[20]

A whole movement developed from Lake's approach, though it appears to operate somewhat at the margins of the disciplines and the church. It included training programs in his methods following a three-tiered approach: (1) church members functioning as carers; (2) clergy, social workers, and teachers operating as professionals; and (3) training in counseling skills. At the core of this training program is personal development with counseling practice and Christian theological reflection. "The pastoral counselor works at the interface between the language of psychology and human behavior, and the language of theology and the knowledge of God."[21]

Inner Healing as Deliverance

In contrast to pastoral counseling is the charismatic healing ministry's emphasis on spiritual inner healing in both the United States and the United Kingdom. These evangelicals are referring quite specifically to the direct work of the Holy Spirit to transform the past to empower people for the present, that is, the healing of memories. The pastor or counselor who is less evangelical, on the other hand, may acknowledge the Spirit's work as giving the strength to the individual to make the necessary changes.[22] A shorthand method of describing these two approaches is that the charismatic emphasizes healing and the therapist focuses on counseling. However, we are trying to avoid precisely this kind of dichotomy and competition in favor of better integration between these fine, yet powerful distinctions.

Duncan rightly condemns the judgmental nature of some evangelical approaches that seems to suggest that unless memories are healed according to their method of deliverance, the healing cannot be authentic. Jesus' position in these matters seems rather clear. When the disciples complained to Jesus that a man who was not one of them was healing in Christ's name, rather than rebuking the man as the disciples expected,

Jesus said, "Do not stop him; for whoever is not against you is for you" (Luke 9:50).

HEALTH CARE AS PREVENTION

Direct health care services include inner healing but also, most important, prevention of illness. An interventionist approach to illness is not enough, but programs of prevention and social reform, which prevent the underlying causes of illness, are necessary. Christian values that eliminate such negative forces as fear, resentment, jealousy, and indulgence can go a long way in creating the psychic climate that can foster good health.

Herbert Benson, a Harvard physician, stated in *Your Maximum Mind* that the faith factor is critical in promoting good health and fighting disease, as was discussed earlier in the Matthews and Dossey material.[23] The church can function as a place of spiritual growth. Through its worship services and prayer groups, it can provide an opportunity for grounding people in God. Believing that we are children of God, forgiven and loved, we will not be as tempted to constantly prove and justify our existence. Being part of a *koinonia* means drug and/or alcohol abuse or other destructive behaviors are no longer needed to mask our loneliness or give us a false high. As we become people who serve others instead of our own needs, we cultivate a healthier approach to life. As we view our bodies as good, to be cared for, we will practice healthier lifestyles.

Preventing Addiction: A Challenge to the Church

Analyzing addiction prevention and treatment is a way of illustrating the church's role in prevention as well as in wholistic treatment. One of the most insidious health problems that undermines physical, emotional, and spiritual health is addiction in all its forms. The church has the responsibility to help its members and others to address the root causes of addiction, thereby helping to prevent its grip on people. This ministry is both a direct service in the prevention mode and a part of long-term educational initiatives. The problem of addiction with its multidimensional nature reflects the importance of the church linking with community, government, and other health care agencies.

Why the Church Should Be Involved

There is a fourfold reason for selecting addiction as an area for the church's attention: (1) addiction is one of the major health care problems in the world; (2) the medical community alone has been unable to meet the full range of people's needs resulting from problems of addiction; (3) the church and its members are uniquely positioned to address the multifaceted issues; and (4) addiction demands by its very nature a collaborative response between church and community.

For the most part the church has not equipped itself to combat addiction, other than its prophetic call for people to love and serve God. In theory this call should be sufficient. In practice, as the prophets learned, all too often it is not. Greater knowledge of and commitment to addressing the devastating problems of addiction are needed, which draw on the full armamentarium of the church's spiritual, human, and financial resources. The church first must engage in self-education on these issues.

Unfortunately, the church has not been extensively involved in the ministry to addicted persons and their families. A 1980 Gallup Poll revealed that only 25 percent of problem drinkers would turn to their church for help; 45 percent of church members responded "no" or "don't know" when asked if they could get help from their clergy about alcohol-related problems.[24] How do illegal drug users feel toward the church; how can the church help them change?[25] Furthermore, there is the perception that drug and alcohol problems are "out there" instead of within our church community. Denial is rampant.

Stephen Apthorp, an Episcopal priest, wrote a highly critical article suggesting that churches are filled with people drastically harmed by alcoholism or drug abuse. However, they cannot be helped by the pastor because he or she has so often come from a family affected by substance abuse that it will be a case of the blind leading the blind. Apthorp went on to say, "No wonder that the church at large and the clergy in particular, have difficulty recognizing and dealing with today's epidemic affliction of addiction. The church and its leaders are clearly among the afflicted, if not the addicted."[26] One of the tragedies of the contemporary church is the myth that if your life is really messed up, you had better stay away from the church because it is for "good" people. Of course, nothing could be farther from the truth since we need God the most precisely when we are in the depths of our greatest sin.

The stories of Scripture and words of Jesus Christ certainly bear out the truth that Christians live as forgiven sinners. Abraham lied that his wife was his sister; David committed adultery; Peter denied Christ; Paul admitted he did the very things he should not. These people were used by God despite their weaknesses. However, the unfortunate fact is that often Christians stand in judgment of other people, giving them a tremendous sense of guilt.

Widespread Patterns of Addiction

Addiction knows no economic, class, race, or cultural boundaries; it is no respecter of persons. Alcoholism and drug addiction are worldwide problems that cut across national boundaries and racial, political, class, and sexual distinctions. In the United States, there is no such thing as a "typical alcoholic." Ninety-seven percent of U.S. alcoholics outwardly are very much like other people, holding down jobs and "getting by" while their inner emotional chaos and physical degeneration wreak havoc on those around them. Only 3 percent of alcoholics in the United States have reached the level of living on the street.

Statistics from the 1970s, 1980s, and 1990s about the widespread nature of alcohol and substance abuse are alarming. Many of the transnational corporations are doing aggressive marketing in developing countries as they experience a decrease of usage in the United States, especially in the use of alcohol. Global alcohol consumption between 1970 and 1977 increased 7 percent in Africa, 11 percent in the Americas, 12 percent in the Eastern Mediterranean, and 25 percent in Southeast Asia. Out of 46 countries with more than a 50 percent increase in beer production and consumption, 42 were underdeveloped countries in the late 1980s.[27] Has the picture improved in the 1990s? Unfortunately, the opposite is the case. "The combined sales of the top 10 global brewers and top 10 distilled spirits companies total nearly $200 billion."[28] A recent study by the World Health Organization, the World Bank, and the Harvard School of Public Health shows that between 3 and 4 percent of all global disease and disability are caused by alcohol. Marketing alcohol consists of targeting the poor, the young, the addicted; encouraging them to drink even more; and capitalizing on local customs as marketing opportunities.[29]

Some specific examples tell the story. Apparently with the Malaysian government's permission, Benedictine D.O.M. (nearly 40 percent alcohol content) touts its "health-enhancing" powers for new mothers with a poster of a woman holding her infant next to a liqueur bottle. In Zimbabwe, where the average income for about 80 percent of people is less than $21 a month, 7 percent of their annual income is spent on alcohol—seven times the proportion spent by U.S. families. The Estonian capital has four times the number of alcohol stores as allowed in most California cities. In 1995, 70 percent of Estonian perpetrators of homicides, serious assaults, and rapes were drunk.[30]

The pervasiveness of substance abuse in the United States is also alarming. During one month in 1997, for example, 200,000 people used heroin; 800,000, amphetamines; 1.5 million, cocaine/crack; 10 million, marijuana; 11 million, alcohol; 61 million, nicotine; and 130 million, caffeine.[31] Among the ten leading causes of death per year, tobacco is number one with 400,000 deaths per year followed by alcohol with 100,000. All illicit drugs combined contributed to 20,000 deaths.[32] Users of drugs, cigarettes, and alcohol comprise one-third of all hospital admissions. The combined medical and social costs of alcohol and other drug abuse were more than $241 billion in 1992, the most recent year for which data is available.[33]

The American Medical Association estimates that in addition to the premature deaths annually attributed to alcohol, the related health, social, and economic consequences of alcohol usage extend far beyond the mortality tables. According to the 1997 Annual Review of Medicine, alcoholism affects nearly 12.5 million Americans and is responsible for annual costs of more than $130 billion from loss of job productivity, deleterious health effects, and direct treatment expenses.[34] Various estimates have shown that 20 percent of suicide victims are alcoholic. Twenty-five percent of persons admitted to general hospitals have alcohol problems. Furthermore, heavy and chronic drinking is the single most important cause of illness and death from liver disease; an estimated 2 to 4 percent of all cancer cases are caused directly or indirectly by alcohol abuse; and 40 percent of all traffic fatalities are alcohol related.[35]

Concern about substance abuse is not only among adults; young people are especially at risk from licit and illicit drugs. Alcohol is the drug most often used by young people, and drinkers are getting younger, according to the 1997 report from the White House Office of National Drug Control Policy. About 9.5 million Americans between ages 12 and 20 had at least one drink in the month preceding the survey; of them 4.4 million were binge drinkers (consuming five or more drinks in a row on a single occasion), including 1.9 million heavy drinkers (consuming five or more drinks on the same occasion on at least five different days).[36] Approximately one in four tenth grade students and one in three twelfth graders report having had five or more drinks on at least one occasion within two weeks of the survey. First use of alcohol typically begins around the age of 13; marijuana around 14.[37]. Alcohol and other drugs are the leading causes of death and injury in teenagers and young adults.[38]

Although drug use has gone down for all but high-risk users in the decades from the 1960s to the 1990s, a crack epidemic in urban areas and the introduction of numerous new drugs mean the dangers of drug abuse are still prevalent. Statistics in 1996 indicated that more than half of all high school seniors have used illicit drugs by the time they graduate.[39] The 1979 peak was 16.3 percent of youth using illicit drugs. "Overall rates of illicit drug use appeared to peak sometime around 1979 and have been decreasing during the 1980s and into the 1990s."[40] A National Household Survey on Drug Abuse, conducted by the Substance Abuse and Mental Health Services Administration in 1993 based on a nationally representative sample of 22,181 people aged twelve and older, revealed that in 1993, alcohol was the most widely used drug for adolescents, cigarettes were second, marijuana was third, and cocaine and inhalants were a distant fourth and fifth.[41] However, marijuana smoking among young people aged twelve to seventeen has nearly doubled since 1992, though the figures are still far below the high reached in 1979.[42]

When asked in 1996 whether they had used marijuana in the past month, almost one in four high school seniors said they had, while less than 10 percent reported using any other illicit drug with the same frequency. Marijuana use among tenth and twelfth graders increased from 40 percent to almost 50 percent lifetime use.[43]

Among the graduating class of 1996, 50.8 percent of students had used an illicit drug by the time they reached their senior year, continuing an upward trend from 40.7 percent in 1992 but still far below the peak of 65.6 percent in 1981. After marijuana, inhalants such as glues, aerosols, and solvents are the second most commonly used illicit drug among young people. Use of LSD (the third most common illicit substance) has gradually increased among eighth, tenth, and twelfth graders each year since 1992. Cocaine use has continued a gradual upward climb but has not reached statistical significance.[44]

Despite a decline in adult smoking, young people in the United States continue to use tobacco at rising rates. In 1996, more than one-third of high school seniors smoked cigarettes, and more than one in five did so daily. These rates are higher than at any time since the 1970s. About 4.5 million American children ages twelve to seventeen now smoke.[45]

The Nature and Process of Addiction

In determining what the church should do, understanding the root causes and process of addiction is the first step. Chemical substances are obvious addictions, but for the church other addictions such as power, stress, or work may dominate. Drug and alcohol misuse cannot be analyzed in isolation from addictive behavior patterns and structures of society. Their underlying causes and links with the fundamental evil in the world, human nature, and our past lives are often overlooked.

Media manipulation and aggressive advertising strongly influence the lifestyle of individuals and communities. Although individual choice is at the core of addiction, there is no doubt that society exerts a strong influence on our decisions. One also has to note the overprescribing of legal drugs, which can be as addictive as anything on the street. Societal goals and individual values, or lack thereof, encourage addictive behavior. Food, sex, tobacco, drugs, and money all become addictions in a society without the proper moral standards.

All addictions have in common a search for pleasure, on the one hand, and an escape from life, on the other; they seek the object rather than its Creator, God. Often it is a form of self-medication used to cope with emotional conflicts and shortcomings. Gerald May defines addiction as "any compulsive, habitual behavior that limits the freedom of human desire."[46] It is caused by the attachment, or nailing, of desire to specific objects. The word "behavior" is especially important in this definition, for it indicates that action is essential to addiction. May describes five essential characteristics of addiction: tolerance, denial, withdrawal symptoms, loss of willpower, and distortion of attention.[47]

Anne Schaef, feminist and psychotherapist, describes two categories of addiction—substance addictions and process addictions.[48] She even goes so far as to state that addiction is any process over which we are powerless. She also describes addictive systems, not just addictive individuals. Substance addictions can be abusing alcohol/drugs, nicotine, caffeine, or food. Food addictions include patterns of binging, purging, or starving, more commonly known as bulimia and anorexia.

Process addictions are addictions to a specific series of actions or interactions. These may include accumulating money, gambling, sex (a way of getting a fix), work (a workaholic uses work to avoid dealing with inner and interpersonal life), stress, religion (Fundamentalists Anonymous is a twelve-step group), or even being addicted to relationships causing judgmentalism, dishonesty, and control of other people.

This addiction to relationships may be expressed in its milder form of expecting another person to meet all our needs.[49] The classic pattern of codependency consists of addiction to another person or to a relationship and its problems. The self-sacrificing person whose own needs are always put last also suffers from an addiction.

Generally, addiction brings to mind addiction to chemical substances because their effects are so rapid and powerful. However, the same kind of cellular dynamics applies to nonsubstance addictions such as gambling, sex, and codependency. There may be different systems of cells, but the patterns of feedback, habituation, and adaptation would be essentially the same.[50]

Addiction to Substances: Its Multifaceted Nature

The multidimensional nature of addiction can be clearly illustrated by examining the characteristics that apply not only to substance abuse but to other addictions as well.

First, it is *physiological*. Alcohol addiction involves a physical predisposition to an illness that includes tissue adaptation, cellular changes, autonomic processes, tolerance changes, and withdrawal reactions. One's genetic makeup can influence alcohol's direct effect on one's persona. Science can now identify at-risk persons, such as children of alcoholics.

Second, there are *psychological* factors: response to stress, conditioning by reward and punishment, compulsive behavior, habit formation, sociocultural conditioning, and denial. The media send covert or hidden messages that feed our psychological attraction to addictions. Peer pressure and low self-esteem can cause us to escape through chemicals. Teenagers, while being warned of the destructive side of crack, PCP, and other drugs, may try them because of the danger or because they have the mistaken notion that they will be immune to their sometimes violent side effects.

The third cause of addiction is *societal*. Anyone who watches television or reads the ads quickly concludes that alcohol provides a lifestyle of fun, sex, and success. However, even more insidious than this glamorization are society's false values. A system where self-centeredness, dishonesty, the illusion of control, and constant crises are the norm must be changed if we are to function as whole and healthy people. A society that emphasizes instant pleasure and material success becomes a breeding ground for drug and alcohol abuse as well as the accompanying crime and carnage.

Fourth, addiction is a *spiritual* problem, a sin against oneself, one's family, and one's community. It is a sin because it destroys the fabric of all three sociologies. It undermines the foundation of human life, which God created.

A 1986 report by the Presbyterian Church (USA), *Alcohol Use and Abuse: The Social and Health Effects*, sums this up very well: addiction is thus a sin in that it (1) is in part individual, (2) is in part collective, and (3) interacts rather uniquely with the drug itself, which plays an increasing role as addiction emerges and progresses.[51] The addict relies, as we all do, upon the grace of God in Jesus Christ. God is at work in the world and in our lives, and we must be well aware of the "log" and "speck" analogy. God's love enables us to regain our self-respect and feel loved while accepting responsibility for the wrong we have done to ourselves and others. Linda Mercadante, for one, argues a sin model of addiction helps both to accept responsibility and to express the gift of God's grace.[52]

How to accept responsibility for our substance abuse while retaining a disease model of addiction challenges treatment specialists. The medical model removes any moral culpability, and the sin model removes a consideration of the physical basis for addiction. The church has a unique opportunity to develop wholistic treatment modalities that recognize the multifaceted nature of addiction.

Behavioral Addictions

Moving from addiction to substances to behavioral addictions, such as stress and workaholism, we see an even more fruitful ground for the church's health ministry. Hans Selye defines stress as "the nonspecific response of the body to a demand."[53] Stress is something that exerts strain or pressure. It may involve happy or unhappy events, pleasant or unpleasant situations. Certain types of stress may be helpful—they may warn us of impending danger or the need to examine parts of our lives that should be changed. Other types of stress are harmful and should be avoided. Stress that is not relieved can do physical damage to the body. Some health care professionals even theorize that illnesses such as asthma, cancer, colitis, and ulcers result from stress.

Research abounds on the causes of stress.[54] Lists of stress factors include changes in lifestyle (from death and divorce, for example); concern over the symptoms of problems; anxiety (at times the cause, at times the effect); depression (at times the cause, at times the effect); marriage conflict; suppression of negative feelings; job; finances; alcohol abuse; smoking; being overweight; nutrition deficiency; excess sugar consumption; allergic reaction; too much caring; lack of socialization; low value system; lack of physical fitness; poor relaxation skills; and low self-worth.

Causes of stress stem first from a lack of self-understanding coupled with low self-esteem.[55] When we accept the church's message that we are unique, special individuals, created in the image of God and loved by God, we regain a sense of self-confidence and worth. We do not need to substitute status or money to booster our feelings of self-worth.

The second cause of stress is workaholism. Persons suffering from low self-esteem may justify their existence by overwork as a type of compensation. The side effects of this kind of driven behavior may be devastating when we claim not to be indispensable but act as if we are. This perception is reinforced by the corporation, church, or other institutions where employers set incredible production and expectation standards. Consider that an estimated 2 to 10 percent of any company's workforce "needs help with a chemical addiction."[56] To some degree, the pressure of the job creates the climate that pushes people to addictive behaviors. Yet employment assistance programs do not tackle this aspect of the problem by changing the adversarial setting or job pressures; they remove people from the setting. A real rehabilitation program would reform the situation that creates addictive patterns.

Part of the root cause of overwork—overprogramming ourselves—does not result only from low self-esteem but can be traced to a distortion of Calvinistic theology, a work ethic or sort of justification by works inherited from our Puritan mothers and fathers. Anne Schaef describes this ethic as workaholism, the designer drug of the church and corporation. Justification by faith and the doctrine of grace may be preached but not lived.

Justification by works stems from a lack of self-esteem where busying ourselves with various projects can push into the background a sense of failure. So workaholism leads full circle to the first cause of stress, lack of self-esteem. Frenetic work produces stress but at its base is a feeling of unworthiness.

A result of workaholism is burnout, an occurrence not only for corporate executives but also for clergy. Reasons for clergy burnout include (1) demands for clergy and her family members to always be role models; (2) reticence of clergy to admit she is unhappy or stressed out; (3) conflicting expectations of a pastor; (4) work to be done exceeds available hours; (5) expectations to increase and keep members even if they are not committed to Christ; and (6) strain of managing emotions, going from funeral to wedding without carrying emotions with her. The pastor begins to feel like a solitary vending machine, dispensing comfort, spirituality, and wisdom as desired by her congregants.

A 1983 study of stress among religious leaders and seminarians was based on sixty-nine persons. They were compared with a population of 201 people in the normative range of stress. Women seminarians experienced more stress than their male counterparts.[57] The study also found that religious professionals are *insignificantly* higher on role overload than the general public. However, in all else, that is, role insufficiency, role ambiguity, role boundary, responsibility, and physical environment, they had less stress and better coping mechanisms.

Stress and overwork are uniformly correlated, but ironically, the opposite of overwork—unemployment—carries its own stress. "Stress and financial hardship created by the economic recession of the early 1970s have had a major impact on illness and death in the United States over the past decade, contributing to as many as 200,000 more deaths than would have been expected," according to a study prepared for the congressional Joint Economic Committee. In addition to financial hardships, lack of meaningful work can cause stress. A study of stress at Hayfield Secondary School in northern Virginia was extremely revealing. The top stressors indicated by students were boredom with classes and too much homework.[58]

A third cause of stress is the loss of a spiritual center and following of false values. Although 90 percent of people in the United States believe in God, this belief does not translate into changed behavior. Is society more stress filled now than in the past? Yes. Is it worse now than for our pioneer ancestors who labored long in the fields? For our ancestors home was home, with no faxes waiting to be answered, no cell phones or e-mails interrupting them. Today people are working even when they are not at the office. Sunday is now a day of sacred shopping.[59] Vacations are no longer times away from the demands of the job.

Herbert Benson has written extensively on the impact of stress on physical and emotional health. The repeated and excessive stress we now experience daily actually creates brain changes.[60] This stems from these false and changing values. Studies have shown that it is not as much the events themselves but the perception of stress and helplessness to face them that is at the root of much of our stress. We have a stress-filled society because our values consist of power, position, and money instead of faith, hope, and love. When we measure ourselves against global standards of achievement in these areas, we always fall short. For example, kids who play Little League baseball end up comparing themselves to World Series players; inflation and pressures for A+ for admission to Harvard or Princeton generate tremendous pressure. Businesspersons view their successes in light of billionaire power brokers such as Bill Gates and Ted Turner. We create unrealistic standards that never allow us to feel a sense of accomplishment and confirm our false belief that we are no good. What we have today is not only Type A personalities but a Type A culture afflicted with what Archibald Hart describes as "hurry sickness."

A *Newsweek* article captured today's mood under the title "Breaking Point."[61] This article recounts how fatigue is now among the top five reasons that people call the doctor. People from Harvard president Neil Rudenstine to a single working mother in California are frayed by the inescapable pressure of technology, frazzled by the lack of time for themselves, their families, their PTAs, and their church groups. They feel caged by their jobs, even as they put in more overtime. The toughest jobs are said to be those of air traffic controllers, doctors, nurses, and secretaries, but experts agree the working mom has the toughest job when domestic chores are not equally shared with a partner.[62] We are fast becoming a nation of the dead-tired. "People are stretched financially, stretched in terms of time and stretched emotionally," says Leah Potts Fisher, codirector of the Center for Work and Family in Berkeley. "So it doesn't take much for them to snap."[63]

Corporations have even coined the category Executive Mach One for someone whose income is over the $100,000 mark. "The accompanying lifestyle necessary for that achievement is simply incredible with a median wake-up time on the fast track at precisely 5:49 a.m."[64] With a schedule like that, burnout is inevitable, leaving one barren of a sense of meaning to life. More than one half of burnout cases that make it into the doctor's office are suffering from depression.

The fourth cause of stress can be other people or life events over which we have no control. We may experience the devastation of a flood or tornado or hurricane, where all our life possessions are swept away; or our only child may be killed by a drunk driver and the feeling of loss and grief fills every corner of our lives, stretching us like a tightly strung rubber band. The overwhelming nature of these events obviously causes stress, depression, and many other mental health problems. At such times the church can be a source of comfort and concrete assistance. Most important, what can the church do to change these patterns that produce stress?

Church Strategies to Combat Addiction

Now that I have outlined the nature and process of addiction and noted its destructiveness, the challenge to the church is how it can *free people from addiction*. A number of strategies have proved effective. They are related especially to the area of substance abuse but are illustrative of what can be done in other areas of stress reduction and other behavioral addictions. These strategies can be implemented by one, several, or a coalition of churches in cooperation with community and government agencies.

Preach, teach, and practice a theology of health, hope, and healing. What is the theological basis for the church's involvement, and what specific methods and programs should it initiate? The first way the church is a resource is by being true to its raison d'être—by preaching a theology of health and hope and providing a caring community.

The theological basis for the church's involvement is not simply concern about the drug problem but is connected to the entire understanding of the church as a health institution and a healing community. Its theology becomes an important tool in combating addiction. Religious values and spiritual perspectives are central resources for preventing and intervening in drug, alcohol, and other problems. The church itself as a caring community is an extension of Christ's healing ministry.

The biblical definitions of health as wholeness and sickness as brokenness reflect health as an integration of body, mind, and spirit—inner and
outer harmony, *shalom*. This view is based on a doctrine of man/woman as
a unified whole. The stewardship of the body is an extension of this integrated view of human nature. There is no dualism in the Bible—health for
the body and salvation for the soul. Health and salvation are twin concepts
signifying wholeness.

We all need restoration, forgiveness, rebirth, and renewal; we are all
broken and suffer from different addictions. Christian theology provides
an analysis of the nature of addiction, its root causes as well as the promise of release. An understanding of the way into addiction helps lead
people out of addiction. Even more important than a theology of health
and sickness, however, is the Christian gospel of hope. Sickness, suffering,
and brokenness do not have the final word. God is in control. God offers
healing in the midst of our brokenness and may use our wounds to heal
us. Henri Nouwen, in his book *The Wounded Healer,* interprets Jesus
Christ's ministry in that light.[65]

Create a caring community of acceptance and a ministry of presence.
Practicing the gospel as a caring community through specific programs is
even more important than preaching. Christ's love motivates people to
become involved in helping others. Preaching the gospel message of forgiveness and restoration is complemented by offering compassion that
leads to a ministry of caring. Prior to launching programs, a caring community of acceptance and forgiveness should be created.

These theological truths form the basis for the current programs to
combat addiction. They provide motivation and understanding of why the
church should be involved. This ministry is not some program tacked on,
not a response from fear or even a sense of service, but is rooted deeply
within the definition of what it means to be a Christian. Christ was a
healer. Christ not only performed healing miracles but also called and
equipped the church to carry forth this health ministry. Ministry to those
with drug and alcohol problems and other addictions is an extension of
Christ's ministry.

As Christians, we do not stand in isolation; we are part of a community—the church. We bear one another's burdens. "He only is whole who
shares in the brokenness of others."[66] Health is not an individual achievement but a community responsibility. We should help move people from
addiction to freedom while creating a climate of acceptance when they fall
short. When people are unable to get help, the church should intervene.
Either its members or the pastor should assist directly or refer them to
someone who can help.

Involvement may mean simple companionship, a covenanting between two people, a presence with a person, an availability. However, this is not a sufficient expression of caring in and of itself. Bringing a person in need into a Christian community is a necessary part of caring. We are created to live in relationship. Isolation and loneliness can cause suffering and even physical illness in the same way as a virus or an accident.

The images of the Christian church in First Corinthians 12, Romans 12, and Ephesians 4 describe the *ecclesia* in terms of a body with many members, a ministry with many callings, a unified spirit with many gifts. The community strengthens who we are as well as defines it. The community has the potential to be a powerful gift of the Spirit. We lose sight of who we were created to be. Alcoholism and drug addiction feed our distorted view of ourselves; our commitment to wrong values; our striving after faulty goals. The community bears witness to Christ, the vision that calls us to affirm our true values and goals. Once alcoholics bring their lives back into accord with God's plan, the odds are in their favor. Life has purpose and meaning. The community also has the power to bring about change that one person alone cannot do. This is a crucial dimension of combating alcoholism and other drug abuse problems.

The theology of compassion and the church as a caring community translate into a ministry of presence, that is, the church in the world. In keeping young people away from drugs we need to be where kids and others gather. That is the principle behind Young Life Clubs, Intervarsity, and other student ministries. The need for positive adult models is central to any values program; curricula are not enough.[67] People are needed who will listen, understand, challenge, encourage, and inspire young people about the possibilities of life, a future where they understand the long-term consequences of their decisions.

This ministry of presence is a need not only with young people who are being tempted but also with the ones doing the tempting—the drug dealers themselves. How seriously does the church take the possibility of conversion? Do we believe that one drug dealer would really give up his lifestyle? Who is the person locked inside the pusher? Since Jesus' ministry was to tax collectors, prostitutes, and thieves, can we do less?

Provide values that encourage healthy lifestyles and positive virtues in our society. A vision of life-affirming, other-regarding ethics is needed where sacrifice for the good of others is the motivator. Sacrificing for long-term positive goals instead of the pleasures of the moment is antithetical to our current instant gratification culture. If goodness, justice, and mercy rule our lives, being good stewards of our bodies while looking past our mere physical health energizes us so that addictive patterns can be put aside.

In the case of pursuing healthy rather than addictive patterns, there are several approaches to curing and preventing addiction: avoidance, abstinence, proper use, and substitution. The application of these solutions depends on the society, the persons, and the substance or habit to which they are addicted.

First, *avoidance*. This is probably better referred to as not getting involved at all. It involves avoiding situations that lead to temptation and subsequent wrongdoing and avoiding participation in destructive addictions.

The other extreme of avoidance, that is, of filling every minute of our lives, also places us in a terribly vulnerable position. When we pursue a workaholic schedule, incredible stress builds, so we seek an outlet and escape through alcohol, drugs, food, or sex. We want these things not for their own pleasure, but as tranquilizers to calm our frantic lives.

Second, *abstinence*. Abstinence probably has received more bad press than any other approach to combat addiction. Since the 1820s, it was many Protestants' approach to alcohol. Fasting is also part of the Christian experience. The second-century Montanists, for example, had periods of abstinence called "dry meals." In the early Middle Ages fish and meat products were occasionally excluded. However, Protestant reformers opposed obligatory fasting as legalistic. In fact, the first formal act of protest in Zurich at the outset of the Reformation in 1522 was a secret banquet of sausages during Lent.

In the Hebrew Scriptures, dietary laws commanded by God were based partially on sanitary grounds and partially on the association of certain foods with pagan rites. In the Christian Scriptures, Paul wrote about the temptations of pagan culture: "It is good not to eat meat or drink wine or doing anything that makes your brother or sister stumble" (Rom. 14:21). Hindus abstain from beef; Jews and Muslims from pork; some Roman Catholics from meat on Friday; Mormons from caffeine; Seventh Day Adventists from all meat.

Abstinence can take two forms: (1) a public policy such as prohibition laws that operated in the United States; or (2) personal avoidance as advocated by Alcoholics Anonymous. In the second instance, an individual's choice need not be extended to others. Even someone who has no alcohol problems can be a witness to others by not drinking.

God created everything in the world and saw that it was good, including the fruit of the vine. All food was for the pleasure and nourishment of humankind. Partaking of wine and other alcoholic beverages as food to be enjoyed is not wrong. However, using them to alter our moods, or escape from ourselves or others, may lead to self-destruction. In the choice of abstinence as a way of dealing with alcohol, for example, the drink itself is not necessarily condemned, but society's or one's inability to control it.

The third approach to potentially harmful substances or actions is *proper use*, that is, of legal substances. The legal nature of a substance is one factor in determining its proper use. Alcohol is socially acceptable, but illegal for certain age groups; marijuana and cocaine are illegal for all, but heroin in the past was used effectively for pain control. Prescription drugs are regularly recommended and dispensed.

Circumstances in which a drug is used make a difference. Valium for the individual suffering from an emotional illness, hospitalization, death of a loved one, or narcotics for the terminally ill cancer patient may be considered justified. The prudence or propriety of using a drug with addictive potential may be very difficult to determine. For example, one may be addicted to sex or work, but both activities when engaged in properly are good, wholesome, and positive. When we become obsessive about them, we no longer apply proper use.

Temperance is the classic virtue that refers to the proper use of potentially harmful substances or actions. For Plato *sophrosune* (soundness of mind) was one of the four cardinal virtues; it became virtually identical with wisdom and justice. For Aristotle *sophrosune* was the mean between self-indulgence and insensibility. Hence, self-control suggests both restraint and mastery of passions and desires.

This virtue was praised in both the Hebrew and the Christian Scriptures. The book of Proverbs had repeated advice about temperate behavior. The pastoral letters echo this same perspective, for example, "Tell the older men to be temperate, serious, prudent, and sound in faith, in love, and in endurance" (Titus 2:2); "And knowledge with self-control, and self-control with endurance, and endurance with godliness" (2 Pet. 1:6).

Thomastic theology combined the biblical perspective with Aristotelian philosophy and viewed temperance as a general and specific virtue. It is a cardinal virtue because the objects of the sense of touch are necessary for human life. The pleasures of touch are natural, and yet it is difficult to control our desires for them. Temperance concerns only the agent, without a direct connection to love of God and neighbor. However, departure from it, for example, sobriety and chastity, may violate love. The reformers, including Calvin, continued the emphasis on moderation. He believed the Scriptures require modesty, contentment with one's lot, patience, and prudence.

The fourth approach is *substitution*. Repeatedly in his letters to Christians in various churches, Paul presented the solution of substitution for sinful and unhealthy life patterns. Galatians 5:19 cites the deeds of the flesh as immorality, impurity, idolatry, jealousy, anger, and drunkenness, among others. The fruits of the Spirit are love, joy, peace, patience, kindness, and faithfulness (Gal. 5:22). The charge of Colossians 3:2 is to set our minds on things above; put aside anger, wrath, and malice; and put *on* the heart of compassion, kindness, humility, forgiveness, and love.

Substitution is the approach used by many who psychologically do not want to admit to an addiction or the explosive nature of their problem. Care must be taken not to replace one addiction with another, for example, alcohol with tobacco or tobacco with food.

The approaches of avoidance, abstinence, proper use, and substitution are important tools in combating addiction, but in and of themselves do not carry the power to transform; this comes from God, faith, and the church.

Develop a systemic understanding of the nature and process of addiction. A systemic approach that recognizes the multifaceted nature of addiction and its underlying causes is crucial for the church as it begins health services to prevent addiction and treat persons with addictions. It cannot work exclusively from a sin model that overlooks the many factors leading to addiction. Without a knowledgeable and educated approach the church can do more harm than good.

A number of things can be suggested from a theological perspective as to the way out of addiction. First, the way out of addiction depends on *transformation*; this is a theological concept even picked up by the secular press. *Metanoia*, that is, conversion, literally means a turning around, a radical change. However, conversion requires the recognition of a need for personal and societal transformation.

Understanding how and why people become addicted is the first step to helping them recover. Paul wrote, "Wretched man that I am! Who will rescue me from this body of death? Thanks be to God through Jesus Christ" (Rom. 7:24–25). What we cannot do by ourselves, God can work in us, the true miracle, the grace of Jesus Christ—what we call transformation.

The beginning of a journey toward wholeness is confessing our sin and accepting Jesus Christ as Sovereign and Savior; however, it is just that, the first step. Simply telling people to accept Jesus Christ is not enough. Help is needed in the daily decisions and approaches that can move people from the slavery of addiction to freedom in Christ, assistance that provides positive alternatives.

The underlying need is a recognition of the problem; denial is the greatest barrier to recovery. Once denial has been overcome, the effect of addiction on oneself, family, and future can be recognized. Desire to change is born out of acknowledgment of adverse effects, but often the desire is to change the side effects rather than let go of the object of the addiction.

Desire to change then leads to an act of the will—to acknowledge one's powerlessness and need of power outside oneself, that is, God—to lead one out of addiction. So in one sense by an act of the will, we acknowledge by the will we cannot change. In theological language, we are in need of God's grace.

The substance, in this case alcohol, may interact with the body, so recovery is not just an act of the will, but is also physiological. For example, at-risk groups such as children of alcoholics who generally have a lower tolerance to alcohol or certain body chemistry may react adversely to small amounts of alcohol, which would not even affect someone else. Of course, there is also the addictive nature of the substance itself, whether caffeine, alcohol, barbiturates, heroin, or cocaine.

Work toward changing economic, social, and racial injustice and false values in society, which create a climate for substance abuse and other addictions. As was discussed previously, the support and advocacy health ministries of the church are important; public policy issues need to be addressed. Many denominations have national lobby and education offices. The United Methodist Church in the late 1980s in recognizing the need to address the climate that fosters addictive lifestyles, especially substance abuse, created Shalom Zones in violent, crime-infested neighborhoods where pushers reigned supreme. This program spearheaded by Bishop Felton May, who was assigned to Washington, D.C., addressed issues of safe, adequate housing, employment, recreation facilities and opportunities and developed prevention programs and curricula grounded in the Christian faith. Methodist and other churches, however, recognized that urban problems were compounded by suburban users who drove their BMWs into the ghettos to get their drugs. False values and injustice are not unique to the urban poor.

Even more effective is *protest*; this method for conducting a war on drugs follows the pattern of the civil rights movement. Martin Luther King's passive resistance or nonviolent protest was both powerful and productive. The support of sheer numbers gathered on the Ellipse, mobilizing the churches, especially African American churches, in the face of mob lynching or the Ku Klux Klan was a vision of what churches and synagogues—the religious community united—can do. It was a voice raised in protest to a society that values money, power, fame, clothes, and prestige over family, friends, service, and honesty; a voice against alcohol and drugs that enslave.

Offer educational programs in prevention for children, youth, adults, and pastors through churches, seminaries, and presbyteries. Such programs were done on a denominational level by the Presbyterian Church (USA). Included in its initiatives were the following:

The *Pastor as Community Organizer*, started in a rural community of six thousand people in the coal mining region of northeastern Pennsylvania, effectively tackled drug problems. Initiated by a Presbyterian minister, it persuaded public and local school authorities to acknowledge the extent of drug use among the community's young people, developed programs of preventive education for youth, and raised public consciousness about drug use and addiction. It developed a coalition among church, school, community, and government.

Training is also an important part of Presbyterian programs. A third of the denomination's synods have held training sessions for presbytery leaders to help them create alcohol and drug awareness programs. In the Synod of the Southwest, a program was established involving every congregation of the synod in active drug/alcohol ministry with special emphasis on work with Native Americans.

The Milford (Michigan) Presbyterian Church played a key part in the formation of a ministry with young people and their families caught in the web of addiction. In rural Georgia, a Presbyterian minister organized a group for Presbyterian professionals who were recovering from addictions. In Jenkintown, Pennsylvania, Grace Presbyterian Church provided office space for a drug abuse counselor who had been ordained by the Presbytery of Philadelphia for this specific ministry. In Two Harbors, Minnesota, the PCUSA has, for some years, been part of a community treatment center that helps recovering addicted people return to a normal life.

National Capital Presbytery Health Ministries, during the 1980s, determined what pastors and educators wanted to learn about substance abuse and presented workshops, consultations, and courses; referred people for treatment; and maintained a resource center. It produced a five-hour video with a study guide, *Organizing the Parish to Confront Problems of Substance Abuse*, and wrote a five-part values curriculum, *Circle of Wholeness*, for parents and teens on the prevention of addiction, which is still being sold.

And at the denominational level, the church estimated that more than half the congregations in the PCUSA have at least studied the issues of drug and alcohol abuse; tens of thousands of copies of a booklet on alcohol and drug awareness resources, *The Congregation: A Community of Care and Healing*, have been sold.[68] In 1978, the Presbyterian Alcohol Network was formed—which later became the Presbyterian Network on Alcohol and Other Drug Abuse and is now part of the Presbyterian Health, Education and Welfare Association (PHEWA)—and provides leadership in this ministry in all synods.

In 1986, a major report, *Alcohol Use and Abuse: The Social and Health Effects, Reports and Recommendations*, was adopted by the General Assembly. The Office of Health Ministries in the Social Justice and Peacemaking Ministry Unit provides information, educational materials, and specialized assistance to congregations, presbyteries, synods, and individuals nationwide. Ten people have been trained as consultants for work with presbyteries and synods in drug/alcohol programs, and are used regularly. A hot line (1-800-325-9133) was established to provide information on alcohol and drug abuse addiction, and confidential help and counseling about treatment. Seed grants for presbytery-based programs have been provided. Pamphlets and other materials have been published, including a sixteen-minute videotape, *Is There an Elephant in Your Sanctuary?*

These impressive programs of the Presbyterian Church are illustrative of what other denominations and church groups are doing as the church proclaims the gospel of Christ, teaching a theology of health, hope, and healing. As the church creates a community of acceptance, witnesses and works in the public arena, and develops realistic and effective programs, it can be part of the answer to the drug problems in our society.[69]

The church is called to be an expression of the gospel, demonstrating redemption and rebirth, spiritual growth, grace, and forgiveness—a corporate good Samaritan. In this regard, the church has a unique role in educating people about the use, nonuse, misuse, and problems of alcohol.[70]

Train intervention teams. Denial, confrontation, and intervention are related concepts. Denial is the biggest roadblock to cure—excuses for why we drink, lies about the amount, failure to see that problems at work are caused by alcoholism rather than the other way around, belief that it is possible to stop at any time, even though we try to and cannot.

Intervention was a method pioneered by the Johnson Institute in Minneapolis. Vernon Johnson recognized the frustration that family members and friends experienced when loved ones did not have the will on their own to seek treatment or stop drinking. The purpose of an intervention was to confront a person with the effects of his or her drinking on others. Often addicts are in such deep denial, they have no idea how destructive their behavior is. Intervention teams are trained to lovingly confront addicts with their destructive behavior, often reenacting various events and the hurt they have caused. These teams most often consist of family members, employees, and friends. A space at a detox and treatment center is arranged ahead of time. The person, if he or she agrees, is taken directly to treatment and hopefully is on the road to recovery.

Develop a congregational, regional, or judicatory policy on substance abuse. Important aspects of developing a policy on substance abuse are the discussion and education by the constituents who form it. The National Capital Presbytery (NCP) policy passed by the Presbytery in January 1991 illustrates this strategy. Unfortunately, few churches are still aware of this policy, which suggests the importance of continuing education about a policy's purpose and application. The purpose of the policy was to provide a foundation for a new understanding of the risks of alcohol and to encourage responsible choices concerning its use. It included the following points: (1) encourage church officers, pastors, and all Presbyterians to incorporate in their daily lives health-giving values in regard to alcohol and to be good role models in their behavior as hosts, family members, church members, and participants in social or business functions, especially discouraging first-time use of beer, wine, and other alcohol by young persons; (2) discourage and challenge heavy drinking in any situation, especially in high-risk situations (for example, during pregnancy or before driving an automobile) and all illegal drinking; (3) support individual abstinence from the use of alcohol as a viable lifestyle in order to promote physical, mental, and spiritual health; (4) encourage, support, and assist individuals suffering from the disease of alcoholism to secure care and treatment; and (5) provide educational programs concerning the use and misuse of alcohol using materials from the Presbyterian, Episcopal, and Methodist Churches and other denominations.

The second part of the policy pertained to local churches. It encouraged them to adopt policies, to take actions to mitigate the potential negative effects of alcohol, and specifically, to consider (1) eliminating the use of alcohol on church property (church property, exclusive of the manse, is herein defined as any building or land owned by the church for its programs); (2) eliminating the use of alcohol at church-related activities (activities using the church's name either on or off church property, or those paid for at church expense); (3) serving grape juice as well as wine at communion; (4) observing alcohol and drug awareness Sunday, the Sunday immediately preceding Thanksgiving, for example, relating information about Alcoholics Anonymous, Al-Anon, Alateen; and (5) making available church facilities for responsible self-help programs (for example, Alcoholics Anonymous, Alateen, and so forth) at minimal cost and working closely with community treatment and counseling programs.

In addition, in recognition that church staff and pastors may become substance abusers, the NCP report encouraged the development of employment assistance programs for church staff who are suffering from addiction, specifically, to (1) encourage the use of the "Clergy Crisis Fund" to augment insurance coverage for treatment/counseling of those seeking to recover from alcoholism; and (2) develop comprehensive health profiles for clergy and other staff designed to identify health risk factors and develop programs designed to assist them in reducing or eliminating these factors.

The third section of the policy promotes public policy and legislative actions, in conjunction with the Social Justice and Peacemaking Unit and the PCUSA Washington Office, to reduce the potential for alcohol misuse, specifically, to (1) reduce the accessibility and advertising of alcohol to persons under the legal drinking age; (2) support more effective penalties for those convicted of driving under the influence or other alcohol-related crimes; (3) protect the public from alcohol-related problems and the resultant violent crimes; and (4) make alcohol less readily available and less attractive, particularly to vulnerable persons, and eliminate the glamorization of drugs and alcohol in the media and advertising.

Advocate laws, policies, and advertising that deglamorize alcohol/drugs and other harmful substances. Drug and alcohol misuse is often analyzed in isolation from addictive behavior patterns and structures of society. The underlying causes and links with the fundamental evil in the world and human nature are overlooked. An essay in *Time* discussed the link between the laissez-faire attitude of the 1960s and the drug epidemic in the 1980s. "In identifying those responsible for the cocaine crisis, President George Bush pointedly included 'everyone who looks the other way.'" Walter Shapiro continues,

> Am I really a fellow traveler in this epidemic of addiction? Do my affectionate, albeit distant, ties to 1960s-style permissiveness render me as culpable as Bennett [Bush's drug czar] claims? Or is my comfortable, middle-class life so far removed from inner-city crack houses and the Colombian drug cartel that any allegation of causal nexus represents little more than politically motivated hyperbole? The honest answer, which both surprises me and makes me squirm, is that to some degree Bennett and Co. are right. My generation, with its all too facile distinctions between soft drugs (marijuana, mild hallucinogens) and hard drugs (heroin and now crack), does share responsibility for creating an environment that legitimized and even, until recently, lionized the cocaine culture.[71]

Media manipulation and aggressive advertising strongly influence the lifestyle of individuals and communities. Although individual choice is at the core of addiction, there is no doubt that society exerts a strong influence on our decisions. Societal goals and lack of positive individual values may encourage addictive behavior. We are living in an age of moral interregnum, where we have used up all the old values without replacing them with new ones; we have sown the wind, and we will reap the whirlwind.

Organize a referral and resource network with community and government agencies and a clearinghouse for materials. Church groups by themselves generally do not have the experience or expertise to collect the large number of resources needed to assist people seeking treatment for addiction problems. Despite fairly rigid church-state separation in face of the terrible drug problems in the United States, this separation was in a sense laid aside with the formation in the late 1990s by the Office of Substance Abuse Prevention (OSAP) of the U.S. government's Interreligious Task Force on Substance Abuse. Representatives of Muslim, Black Muslim, Buddhist, American Indian, Roman Catholic, Protestant, Jewish, and several independent religious groups from various racial and ethnic perspectives met together; our pooling of curricula, prevention materials, strategies, and programs enriched and expanded our own individual capacities to address drug/alcohol problems within our respective communities.

Often referral systems are more modest. Individual pastors, for example, may visit community agencies, treatment programs, rehabilitation centers, and health care professionals who work in this field. Cecil Williams, pastor of Glide Memorial Church in San Francisco, followed this pattern.[72] Pastors often develop their own networks both to keep informed in the addiction field and to develop resources to share with others.

Organize and participate in ecumenical coalitions to combat substance abuse, domestic violence, and other addictions including international information networks on production, distribution, and use. Experience indicates that the most effective ecumenical and interfaith programs are born out of cooperative endeavors to meet recognized needs. That is certainly the experience in the substance abuse field. I was part of an Interfaith Coalition in the late 1980s in Washington, D.C., "Just Say No to Drugs." Thus I can testify firsthand that theological differences were laid aside and solutions achieved by Muslims, Jews, Protestants, and Catholics working together to overcome the common enemy of drug-related violence in the nation's capital. The money and power of the drug lords could be confronted only by a united front of no toleration.

This initiative included not only recognized leaders of the above religious groups and addiction treatment specialists but also local people whose neighborhoods were being decimated. An interreligious initiative has several advantages: (1) smaller congregations can be involved who by themselves could not sustain a program; (2) collective wisdom on strategies provides a broader base for program support; (3) financial support can be shared across a larger constituency; and (4) a united initiative provides more political power with a greater possibility of success on a long-term basis. One caution is in order. Interfaith programs can become so broad that no one group feels ownership or responsibility. First, the individual groups need to be strong and experienced to ensure collective success.

This examination of some details of specific church-based health care in the prevention, intervention, and treatment of addiction indicates the need for a model for church involvement in other health-related issues. In conclusion, the church has a unique opportunity with the failure of our health care system to redefine and implement new health care practices and programs. By redefining health, it sets forth a broader agenda for health care delivery where needs of the body, mind, and spirit are attended as well as aggressive initiatives for prevention of sickness and suffering.

8

Parish Nursing—a New Specialty

Although the church has been involved for centuries in a health and healing ministry, as indicated in chapter 1, now is the fullness of time for the church to develop new directions for its health ministries. The parish nurse movement has had a tremendous impact in the late 1980s and 1990s in helping congregations to begin a health ministry and provide the necessary leadership. Hence, it is important to understand something about it and how a parish nurse may revitalize a church's mission in health.

The experience and vision of these new health ministers are truly amazing. They collectively represent a large cross-section of the church in terms of age, geography, theology and, to some extent, racial-ethnic background. The energy, commitment, and vibrant faith are contagious. The annual Westberg Symposium sponsored by the International Parish Nurse Resource Center focuses on creative worship and an inspiring exchange of ideas.

The significance of the parish nurse has been documented in numerous sources. It is perhaps the fastest growing specialty within nursing today. The movement was conceptualized by Rev. Granger Westberg, a Lutheran clergyman. Parish nursing is a professional model of health ministry with the health minister being a registered professional nurse. A health minister does not have to be a parish nurse because it is a broader term inclusive of other disciplines. Here the focus is more narrowly on the parish nurse.

What follows is not a definitive description of parish nursing but some impressions based on personal experience over the past fifteen years.[1] In the mid-1980s as director of National Capital Presbytery Health Ministries, I wrote parish nurse job descriptions; cohosted a television special in Washington, D.C., in 1990 on the subject; discussed parish nursing in my courses and lectures on health ministry; and was involved in setting up some of the early training programs. These experiences are supplemented by a review of the body of literature on the subject, conversations with health care professionals and pastors in the United States and the United Kingdom, and travel with my research assistant, Jane Ferguson, to selected parish nursing sites on the East and West Coasts of the United States.

SPECIALIZATION IN NURSING

The development of this new nursing specialty follows that of the clinical nurse specialist, which is recognized as a profession and legal designation for advanced nursing practice. The growth of nursing as a profession accelerated after World War I, necessitating differentiation and specialization. Specialization first occurred informally as nurses selected specific areas for practice and, through independent study and practice, became knowledgeable and skillful in caring for persons with specific needs.

Role definition is achieved through the development of norms, attitudes, standards, and new expectations that must be integrated through observation and participation. In the early years of parish nursing, since there were only a handful of nurses practicing this yet-to-be-designated specialty, a source to assist in role definition was the Parish Nurse Resource Center. The center was founded for the purpose of taking that learning of the original six parish nurses, the congregations they served, and Lutheran General Hospital, the partnering hospital, and making this learning available to all interested parties. One group of interest was the clinical nurse specialist (CNS). Some have cited it as an illustration of how nursing specialties began, which helps us to understand parish nursing.[2]

After World War II, Hildegard Peplau recognized the need for formal advanced preparation for clinical specialists and started the first clinical nurse specialist graduate program at Rutgers University in 1954.[3] She cited three reasons for initiating the clinical nurse specialist role: (1) increased knowledge germane to the field of specialization; (2) development of new technology; and (3) response to a hitherto unrecognized public need or interest. Sociological literature cites that changes in the complementary characteristics of a system or roles (such as in the health care system) are stimulated by technology, increased organizational complexity, and new output demands. Role differentiation implies the reallocation of existing role expectations to meet new organizational expectations.[4] The parish nurse movement is responding to these professional and sociological criteria for instituting a new nursing role, as well as being grounded in the theological framework described earlier.

The evolution of a new specialty has predictable and observable phases: role identification and differentiation, role definition, setting standards, educational preparation, justification, and certification. Most current nursing specialties have passed through these phases, but not all have followed this sequence.

DEVELOPMENT OF THE PARISH NURSE SPECIALTY

Identification of a new role develops from the "soil of social organization."[5] The "soil" that has fostered the germination of the parish nurse role has been the need for an integrated approach to health and healing in response to soaring health care costs, a decrease in the overall health of the nation, and the absence of the religious community, especially the church, in health care. The increased health costs result from, among other factors, medical advances and increased technology, which prevent death from acute illness but do little to promote healthy lifestyles that prevent acute and chronic disease and injury. (See chapter 2 for further discussion of this point.) The key to improving health lies with the individual and his or her lifestyle choices and in society's need to provide a safe and healthy environment. These issues are best addressed from the whole person definition of health and the responsibility of each individual to be a "good steward" of one's body. This also includes being one's brother's or sister's keeper in the areas that affect the abilities of others to fulfill their health potential.

History of Parish Nursing

The historical roots of parish nursing stem from several sources. First, the early work of the Nurses Christian Fellowship by members such as Shelly Fish, Ruth Stoll, Norma Small, and others who affirmed the appropriate role of the nurse in the spiritual dimensions of health. The spiritual wellness inventory developed for use by nurses was one of the earliest instruments of its kind based on an integrated understanding of what constitutes health.

Second, as mentioned previously, the work of Granger Westberg in the 1960s in founding Wholistic Health Centers for primary health care, which included pastors, family practitioners, social workers, and nurses as a health team, created the aegis for parish nursing. Since the nurse was recognized as the health professional who most often held the team together, by the 1980s when economics and practicality inhibited the expansion of these Wholistic Centers, the idea of parish nurses was born. It began ecumenically in hospitals and parishes, and embraces an interfaith style.

Third, the black Baptist and Pentecostal churches' "church nurse" contributed to the historical precedent for the two terms coming together. The church nurse, who was not a trained nurse, was quite limited in her functions, for example, reviving those "slain in the spirit" with smelling salts—ministering to members becoming ill during a service. The fact that these churches recognized the church nurse in a generic sense as a part of the ministerial staff was an important contribution, though it was a non-professional nurse model.

In addition, deaconess nursing in Kaiserwerth, Germany, and Scandinavia through the Lutheran Church provided a model of parish nursing in the early 1800s that is still flourishing.

> Some schools, including the Lahti College of Parish Social Services in Lahti, Finland, incorporate diaconal education into the basic baccalaureate nursing curriculum. The curriculum at Lahti includes courses in parish social services, theology, ethics, caring science and caring theology. Diaconal studies are also available at the graduate level in both Norway and Finland. For twenty years the deaconesses were the only nurses in Norway. As the century turned, about 400 of them worked in various capacities.[6]

The most recent phase of parish nurse development is the establishment of the International Parish Nurse Resource Center and the publication of the *Parish Nurse Newsletter* and numerous books and articles. With experienced and strong leadership this center has provided the resources needed for such a fast-growing movement. It is now under the umbrella of Advocate Health Care, and its crucial place is (hopefully) secured. In addition, the founding of a national Health Ministries Association, a professional organization for parish nurses and other health ministers, testifies to the importance of parish nurses.

The parish nurse movement is timely as health care changes its main venue from the hospital to the community. The technological focus of the medical model has meant that medicine has mainly been practiced in the hospital setting for much of this century. But as managed care makes hospitals less profitable, the focus is moving to preventive health in the community, including the church.

With increased awareness that lifestyle is a personal responsibility, people are encouraged to take an active role in promoting their own health by learning more about health and illness and by practicing self-care behaviors, such as diet modification, exercise, and stress reduction. These activities are largely outside the formal health care institutions and health care reimbursement systems. They appropriately should be assumed within the mission of faith communities with their theological mandate to promote wholeness in the image of God and their breadth and depth in reaching all age, socioeconomic, racial, and ethnic segments of society.

The need for parish nurses is evident from their rapid growth in numbers from a handful in 1984 to more than 2,000 today.[7] The national Health Ministries Association has more than 650 parish nurses on its mailing list. In 1984 there were only 6 nurses working in six congregations— two Roman Catholic churches, and four Lutheran and Methodist churches.[8] How carving out this role from within and without the current health care system will impact on other legally and ethically defined healing roles, health institutions, including the church, and the health care system is part of the future questions.

Parish Nursing—a New Specialty

A reenvisioned understanding of health propels the church to an enhanced role in a health and healing ministry. The parish nurse is the best professional to help the church assume its central role. Nursing, which prepares and socializes its members into a whole-person, health-promotion, continuing-care-practice model, is the profession best prepared to integrate health and wholeness into the faith community's worship, education, and ministry. This is a practical way of including the church as a part of the health care system. Specifying a parish nurse signifies that she is not just a generic nurse located in a church but one who has additional nursing knowledge and skills and theological understanding of health and wholeness. Defining the role of the parish nurse and implementing this new concept have been the challenges facing the parish nurse movement today.

The American Nurses Association (ANA) in 1997 recognized parish nursing as a specialized practice of professional nursing, and the ANA adopted the *Scope* and acknowledged the *Standards of Parish Nursing Practice*. On the one hand, the definition of the parish nurse role is broad enough in scope to encompass the diversity in size, location, composition, and values of faith communities in which the parish nurse role may be implemented. The parish nurse is more than a community health nurse. On the other hand, in order to achieve clear identity and acceptance within the professional and health care communities, the definition is specific enough to allay territorial concerns of other specialties as well as give a clear picture to the consumers and employers of their expectations concerning investment of time and the church's resources. Parish nurses can only do the independent practice of nursing for which they are licensed.

The uniqueness of parish nursing is its focus on the faith community, its members (families and individuals), and its ministry to the larger community. Several excellent curriculum models have been developed by the International Parish Nurse Resource Center and other institutions to address this scope of practice.[9]

Now that the specialty is defined and standards of practice developed, it must be justified through research based on practice and health outcomes. While we would like to think that the concept and goals of parish nursing are sufficient to secure economic support, even faith communities must translate their faith into economic reality. By means of analyzing cost-benefit ratios and measuring outcomes, churches can be good stewards of the resources entrusted to them by their members. Sources for funding of parish nurses are emerging as an important topic as their contribution is becoming more and more valued.

The last phase in a new specialty is attaining national recognition of the expertise demonstrated by practitioners of the role. In nursing this process, called professional certification, requires the demonstration of advanced knowledge and skill beyond the competent standards of the practice. The criteria for professional certification may be established by the American Nurses Association or other nursing specialty organizations and require a certification examination in addition to education and practice criteria. The next step will be developing a certification examination, but the cost, estimated to be $100,000, is currently inhibiting this step. Professional certification is frequently confused with "institutional certification." Institutional certification is established by an institution such as a denomination or health care agency to insure the qualification of those practices within the institution (such as clergy). These criteria may be standards of care and/or professional performance that are higher than the "competent" standards of practice recognized by the profession, but may not be recognized nationally as professional certification, the mark of excellence.

Now that the parish nurse has been accepted as legitimate within the profession of nursing, it must be embraced by the health care system, which includes the church, community agencies, and acute long-term care institutions. The task of defining and interpreting the parish nurse's role in relation to other healers and to the clients it will serve is crucial to role implementation.

The International Parish Nurse Resource Center has facilitated the definition process through its networking functions, annual meetings, curriculum, and resource materials and help in launching the organization of the Health Ministries Association (HMA). As the preparation of nurses for the parish nurse specialty has become more formalized, their role is even more crucial. The HMA, which expanded from several dozen members at its organizational meeting in 1989 to more than a thousand members in 1999, both provides a society to establish educational standards and serves as a professional membership organization. This may foster more cohesion within the specialty in the future.

From the norms and attitudes that have evolved thus far, identification of competencies has been determined so that education programs, whether continuing education or academic, can be developed. There has been extensive discussion about the need for a formal degree program versus continuing education to be a parish nurse. I was involved in piloting a master of arts in parish nursing at the Georgetown University School of Nursing in the mid-1980s, but the costs and time required to complete the degree made it prohibitive for nurses. These questions are being more and more debated but are not yet resolved. However, those calling themselves parish nurses are required by the "Standards of Professional Performance" to acquire the knowledge and skills to meet the competency level of the "Standard of Care."

Profile of a Parish Nurse

Parish nurses typically feel "called" to their profession, articulating the need to use the gifts God gave them by incorporating their faith with their healing profession. In the age of managed care, parish nursing offers a welcome relief to the mechanization and bureaucratization of health care. "One of the reasons we enjoyed parish nursing so much was that we didn't have to spend so much time with paperwork," remembers one seasoned parish nurse. "We had the freedom to 'be' with people in their joy and pain, and not be locked into time-consuming documentation."[10]

Parish nurses are registered professional nurses. They come to churches with different stories. Some are retired. Some are burned out by the medical profession after years of working in intensive care units. Others, in states where social services have been cut, are hard-pressed to find work in hospitals upon graduation from nursing school, and look to churches as an alternative source of employment. Still others have started to raise a family and are interested in part-time work. Common to all is a religious faith they bring to bear on the healing art they practice.

The parish nurse may be a member of the church she or he serves. When the church has not had a nurse to draw from its ranks, it has found that having a nurse who is not a member of the church, or even the same denomination, can be beneficial. Sometimes church members talk more comfortably about their concerns to a parish nurse who is not a church member because they are less worried about confidentiality.

Overwhelmingly, parish nurses are women. They range in age from their twenties, if they have just graduated from nursing school, to their sixties, if they are retired. Most parish nurses are of a mature age, more spiritually seasoned than younger nurses, who naturally tend to be more ambitious, eager to acquire new skills and advance in their profession.

In an age of malpractice suits and criticism of managed care, the parish nurse blows as a fresh wind or one might even say the breath of the Holy Spirit, offering compassionate care and nursing competence. The caring style of the parish nurse engenders confidence and trust on the part of parishioners, which may not exist between professional and patient in other avenues of the health care system. This spontaneous, wholistic approach to health, enhanced by the movement of the Holy Spirit, is the province of the parish nurse and signals what is missing in the current health care system. She or he can provide the catalyst for the church to rediscover its unique healing ministry. Granger Westberg, the pioneer of parish nursing, observed,

> A congregation willing to test out the idea of a parish nurse on their staff soon learns that this is an entirely new kind of nurse. She has entered this kind of nursing because she is convinced that traditional nursing makes it difficult for a spiritually motivated nurse to treat her patients holistically. Hospital protocol keeps her very busy doing mechanical kinds of good deeds, leaving no time for a listening ministry—to say nothing of a teaching ministry in which the Christian way of life can be understood as health enhancing.[11]

The distinguishing characteristic of nursing is its emphasis on care, not just cure, and on prevention through health education. Parish nursing forms the bridge between the medical establishment and the church/synagogue. Indeed parish nurses find they must listen with a "third ear" to detect the deeper spiritual wound that may be behind a congregant's stated physical complaint. The calling card may be that the "scratch is getting red," but the parish nurse soon finds herself listening to problems about the person's marriage, stress at work, or sadness and depression. Her wholistic approach, which embraces a concern for body, mind, and spirit, offers the opportunity to uncover the deeper issues some people might be too intimidated to announce to the pastor or even admit to themselves.

Whereas most nurses usually see patients only when they are ill, the parish nurse sees congregants over a continuum of good times and bad, so she has a keener sense of when intervention is needed. In time of crisis, when a mother is grieving the loss of a child, the parish nurse is there to remind the mother to drink lots of water, the simple health habits a traumatized individual forgets and a pastor may overlook. By encouraging congregants to take care of their physical needs, the parish nurse helps them rally their own spiritual forces to deal with a crisis. She reminds people they have a body when they are in spiritual crisis and links them to the spiritual realm during times of physical illness.

Qualifications for Parish Nurses

The qualifications to be a parish nurse are partly related to the job description or self-defined role that she assumes. Her roles obviously affect the necessary qualifications. Generally, to date there has not been much rigor in required qualifications. In many cases being a registered nurse with a desire to work in a church either in a paid or in a volunteer capacity is considered sufficient. However, now that the scope and standards of parish nursing have been developed, that situation will change.[12]

The eight standards of professional performance, as set forth by the Health Ministries Association, accompany what one would generally expect from nurses including proposed measurement criteria.[13] They cover quality of care, performance appraisal, education, teaching and sharing with colleagues, respecting of values and beliefs of others following professional ethics, collaboration with agencies and other health providers, continued research on parish nursing practice, and utilization of effective resources to achieve desired outcomes.

Early on, Iowa Lutheran Hospital spelled out several qualifications necessary for a parish nurse as it initiated positions and training in this new specialty:

The first qualification relates to *education*. The person should be a registered professional nurse with a current nursing license, BSN or RN, and active in a continuing education program relating to parish nurse responsibilities. David Carlson, Director of Parish Nursing, Meriter Hospital, Madison, Wisconsin, recognized this opportunity in the way his training programs were established when he was at Iowa Lutheran Hospital. He stressed the "pastoral model" rather than a "medical model." This experience-based education program is one year in length.

It begins with three weeks of intensive clinical pastoral education at the hospital, followed by an internship in a congregation(s). During the internship the candidate returns at regular intervals to Iowa Lutheran Hospital for seminars and collegial interchange. The curriculum seeks to develop competencies in pastoral care, community health nursing, wholistic health and wellness, psychological concepts, assertiveness training, and marketing and salesmanship.[14]

Second, in terms of *experience*, three to five years of nursing experience were suggested as a minimal standard, preferably in one or more of the following areas: public health, education, public schools, medical/surgical nursing, and/or emergency room outpatient nursing.

Third, the category of *personal* qualifications received the greatest emphasis. These included a broad range of qualifications: knowledge of healing/health ministry of the church; the practice of wholistic health philosophy; skill in communication and teaching techniques; knowledge in health promotion and of health services and resources in the community, including public health and hospice; motivation to grow personally and professionally with a knowledge of current nursing and health care issues; participation in church and community activities that contribute to professional growth and to the promotion of wholistic philosophy; knowledge of and compliance with the Code of Ethics of Nursing and the Nurse Practice Act of Iowa, including the practice of confidentiality and professional standards; membership in professional organizations; and individualized study programs. In addition, they suggested that a person should be willing to donate time as a parish nurse for a year with the possibility that the church would consider making the parish nurse a salaried person after a one-year pilot project.[15]

Salary of a Parish Nurse

The salary, unlike that of other professions, is correlated not with years of experience or training but with the available funds for these newly created positions. Funding for parish nursing is available through some church denominations, resulting in a church-based health ministry. But many hospitals also are eager to fund hospital-based parish nursing programs in churches. The hours and pay for parish nurses vary. Some work from five hours to twenty hours a week at the rate of roughly twenty dollars an hour. Others who are not sponsored by hospitals volunteer for the first few years; later their church may start paying them. However, if a volunteer parish nurse is doing an effective job, a congregation may realize her importance only after she leaves and not recognize the need for financial support. The majority of parish nurses still work as unpaid staff.

STYLE OF PARISH NURSING

Not only because it is a new specialty but also because of the grassroots development of the ministry, parish nurses must be flexible. Some have church offices with regular hours. Others prefer to go where the parishioners are, in their homes, at their church committee meetings, or after services on Sunday. One parish nurse began with office hours and found that no one came, so she went to the Sunday coffee hours, attended women's meetings, and started a Bible study group. Usually, the parish nurse combines office hours with a roving visitation schedule in the community.

Parish nurses network by going to parish nurse support groups organized either by the hospitals that sponsor them or by the Health Ministries Association chapter in their area. There they swap ideas and help one another solve problems they have encountered in their ministry. Parish nurses assert that the uniqueness of each program leads to collegiality. It is important that parish nursing continues to reflect individuality and creativity in its different styles that meet the local needs.

There is no such thing as a typical day in the life of a parish nurse. Unhampered by the exigencies of bureaucracy, parish nurses operate with a flexibility that allows them to respond to the moment. Consider, for example, the parish nurse who was called upon to distribute communion to a depressed and homebound elderly mother of five grown children who were their mother's caretakers. Taking the time to talk to the weeping mother, the parish nurse discovered that the source of the elderly woman's depression was a power struggle between her and her children. Much to her children's distress, she was refusing to take the medication that was keeping her alive because as she saw it, her children were trying to force the medicine on her without respecting her desire not to take it. The parish nurse observed the psychological dynamics of an elderly woman unwilling to give up control to her children because of her pride and the deeper spiritual wounds caused by her feeling that her children no longer respected her. Acting on her medical knowledge, the parish nurse was able to determine that three of the four pills the mother was taking were essential for her life; the fourth pill was a painkiller that the mother could decide whether she wanted or not: giving the mother the choice to take this last pill gave back her self-respect. The parish nurse then did a role-play to teach the mother and the daughter how to communicate in a respectful way through listening and paraphrasing to each other what they had said in order to let the other know she had been heard.

Parish Nurse as Initiator of Health Ministry

Sometimes the parish nurse is a catalyst for a health ministry within her or his church, and at other times the needs of the church dictate the type of health ministry that unfolds. In some cases, a hospital will launch a parish nurse program in a church and provide financial support under community outreach before the church builds a budget for the program. Hospitals have found parish nurses to be much more effective in teaching preventive health than any mass marketing campaign. The parish nurse builds trust with patients and visits them one-on-one in their homes and in the church, where people feel safe and comfortable. It is not unusual to find a nucleus of interdenominational and even interfaith groups supported by a local hospital to implement a parish nursing program.

At one parish nurse support group sponsored by a local hospital, a salesperson for a health care company was there to promote the sale of a remote calling device for use by elderly persons in their homes to alert their families and the medical establishment for help in case they fell or were disabled. The danger of some hospitals' enthusiasm to launch parish nurse programs in churches as a way to market to their clients in the community is that they might be too overeager. Churches may take on parish nursing before they have had time to lay the groundwork for a health ministry program into which the parish nurse fits. However, this may be a moot point, considering that health ministries are often sparked by the startup of a parish nurse program or at least simultaneous with it.

The churches may also launch parish nurse programs and then lodge them in the community after they have gained acceptance. When parish nurses start a health ministry program at their church, they ideally approach the pastor and church council armed with facts and an argument. They define health ministry and explain how it fills the gaps of the U.S. health care system, which has fewer financial resources and time to care for the poor, the elderly, and the unemployed. They point out that the majority of health care problems can be adjusted by lifestyle changes—a natural niche for the church. They quote Scripture that calls the disciples of Christ to address health. They speak of the need for advocacy, especially for the elderly who find the present health care system exceedingly complicated and difficult to negotiate. They present the idea of bringing the concept of the unity of body, mind, and spirit to the congregation. They can help to reenvision good health as a community responsibility, not an individual achievement, and propose a health ministry/parish nurse program supported by a commission of selected members from the congregation (including the pastor) who would serve as advisors to the parish nurse and evaluate her activities.

In many cases, parish nurse proposals have been enthusiastically accepted by the church governing body, but on occasion they are rejected. Confident in her call, one parish nurse whose request had been spurned asked the church to let her volunteer for six months, and then the church could decide whether to support a health ministry or not. The church was completely won over after six months, and has been operating a thriving health ministries program for several years. In other cases, the nurse's ideas are readily accepted because the pastor is already aware of the benefits of the whole person health approach because she has practiced alternative healing techniques before becoming a pastor.

Pastor and Parish Nurse Collaboration

It is crucial for a parish nurse to be part of the church staff in order to give her credibility with the congregation: committees may come and go, but a staff member is viewed more seriously. A parish nurse knows she has arrived when her name is listed under the names of the pastor and the deacons in the church bulletin and on the church letterhead. Some parish nurses meet with the pastor on a weekly basis, especially to discuss whom they have visited, and attend staff meetings and retreats. Together they decide the course of action, working as a team to try to bring a person to a healthier place both spiritually and physically. As a team, the pastor and the parish nurse can ride on each other's coattails: if the parish nurse sees a patient she thinks is in need of deeper spiritual direction than she is equipped to provide, she alerts the pastor; if after a home visit the pastor is concerned that a person is not receiving proper care, or has a physical ailment, the pastor can call the situation to the attention of the parish nurse.

This need for a collaborative style was precisely the motivating factor to start a parish nursing program at one church in Pennsylvania where the pastor was making regular visits to a homebound church member only to discover that she was missing the cues of the church member's failing eyesight, which signaled advanced diabetes. The church member needed her legs amputated because of her untreated diabetes, a situation that might have been prevented had a parish nurse been on staff to recognize the red flags. However, it is not always the parish nurse who saves the day.

The pastor can offer the parish nurse perspective on what it means to heal, curbing the nurse's desire to cure and helping her negotiate the thorny theodicy questions. When the physician can do no more to heal the ill person, the task for caring for the patient is not over. As the patient struggles to adapt to limitations and pain, the parish nurse and the pastor are there to assist in that adaptation. In the face of suffering, all healers need one another's support. The doctor who pronounces the illness to be incurable, the patient who must adjust to the news, the parish nurse who cares, and the pastor who prays for healing are equally in need of God's grace. The key element that separates the parish nurse from other public health or community health educators may be her freedom within the religious community to emphasize and enhance the spiritual dimensions of health. At that point the cooperation between the parish nurse and the pastor is most fruitful.

The Parish Nurse as Part of the Health Care Team

The parish nurse does not do all of this work by herself. Though a nurse might be approached by the pastor to handle all the suffering and grief-stricken people in the church by herself, the wise pastor and parish nurse know that it takes a team to make a health ministry work; one person would be crushed by the challenge. Ideally, a parish nurse is part of an overall health ministries program. The standards of practice define her clients as the faith community, a family and the individual. There might be several health ministry programs in addition to parish nursing, such as grief support groups, parenting support groups, healing liturgies, and home visitation. Each group has a volunteer leader from the congregation who enlists the volunteers for that group.

The parish nurse is the glue that holds the health ministry program together by offering support and training to volunteer leaders and their volunteer recruits. For example, as part of the goal to integrate health into the spiritual teaching of the church, the parish nurse may need to work closely with the Christian educator. Her goal is to integrate health and wholeness concepts into the existing curriculum for all ages as well as to arrange special education programs dealing with specific problems such as teenage pregnancy. If the Christian education director perceives the parish nurse as competition for time and resources, the collaboration may be inhibited unless the director is knowledgeable about the overall health ministry team.

Since promoting self-care requires health education about diet and medication, professional nutritionists and pharmacists may feel that clients should come to them instead of the parish nurse for this information. Incorporating members of the congregation with health-related expertise into the health and healing program will not only enrich the program but also provide another source of integration rather than conflict. The role of the parish nurse must be well defined as integrating spiritual aspects of health and healing with the noninvasive, medical functions of nursing as prescribed by state regulation, lest physicians and nurses in the community become wary that the parish nurse will "take away their patients." Enlisting physicians and nurses in the congregation to help interpret the parish nurse role to community physicians may allay their fears.

Promotion of self-care and a whole person approach to health is viewed by some professionals in the medical community as antiphysician. But it is less threatening when viewed as the ethical right and spiritual responsibility of an individual to be informed and to make choices about health and health care according to a person's level of development and ability. The intervention by others when there is a deficit in self-care may reassure physicians that people needing medical diagnosis and treatment will be referred as appropriate. The parish nurse must know her limits and refer to specialists and qualified practitioners when the resources are not available within the congregation. In case management and referral of individuals and families the parish nurse may be perceived as infringing on the domain of the social worker. Once more, collaboration is the ideal in order to help the members of the congregation to reach their highest level of self-care in their journey toward wholeness.

Though a church can have a health ministries program without a parish nurse, or vice versa, churches may find each is weakened by the loss of the other. Without a health ministries program and a cabinet, the parish nurse finds it difficult to get the support she needs; without a parish nurse, the church misses out on the professional expertise the nurse affords the programs. Usually, the parish nurse reports to a health ministry committee, which may be organized according to the polity of the church into a commission, a committee, or a cabinet. At a United Church of Christ program, for example, the parish nurse first reported to a Mission and Service Commission but became so successful that a Health Ministry Commission was formed all on its own with a seat on the church governing body.

THE FUNCTIONS OF PARISH NURSES

There are an expanding number of models and functions of parish nursing. They range from an empowerment for health model to direct health care services, such as the measurement of blood pressure, to preventive, educational approaches. Parish nurses generally follow a preventive rather than a crisis model. A referral system is especially important for the maximum use of a parish nurse. She can fulfill various functions, enriching the church's health ministry and serving the health needs of the community.

Parish nurses typically offer services that fall into the seven categories of advocacy, empowerment, prevention, training, personal health counseling, liturgical, and direct health care services, described below.[16] Besides these activities, the parish nurse organizes church health fairs where congregants can go from booth to booth and get anything from flu shots, a cholesterol screening, or a foot massage. To help with large events such as health fairs and home visitation programs, the parish nurse draws on the doctors, nurses, and wholistic practitioners who are members of the church and are willing to volunteer their time. At one of these health fairs, the pastor of one church attended a booth offering stroke awareness in order to encourage parishioners to do the same. During the course of the screening, he discovered he had an atrial fibrillation, which prompted him to seek further testing that revealed he was heading for a stroke. Medication was prescribed along with a change in lifestyle that resulted in a loss of thirty pounds. He informed the parish nurse that he had renewed energy and felt better than he had in ages, an example that the parish nurse can serve an essential purpose by saving the life of the church pastor!

The functions described here reflect the variety of activities in which a parish nurse may be involved, although not every parish nurse offers all of these services since the congregation determines the needs. Sometimes these categories overlap. In advocating for parishioners, for example, a parish nurse models what people have the right to demand of a doctor, thus empowering them to stand up for themselves in the future.

Advocate

Often, parish nurses will advocate for the elderly or newly arrived immigrants in their congregation who have difficulty with English as they try to wend their way through the cumbersome and often complicated corridors of the medical establishment. Parish nurses will accompany parishioners into the doctor's office and explain what the doctor is prescribing. In many instances, parish nurses are able to secure patients extended stays in the hospital, occupational therapists, or a health care worker to take care of them at home. Because of their medical vocabulary and knowledge of how the system works, they are effective in accessing the health care system. In many ways, they bridge the gap between the health care system and the patient.

Parish nurses may be advocates for the family of a patient. For example, a wife who could not get her husband to go to the doctor asked him to see the parish nurse, and she was able to persuade the man to visit a physician. On a broader level, parish nurses may help the church advocate the rights of mentally ill or disabled persons or others in the community marginalized by their health condition.

Functional and ethical aspects of the advocacy role may bring the parish nurse into conflict with some physicians. Physicians may not welcome the parish nurse's flagging undetected health problems or changes in health status that they missed. Unresponsiveness by a physician may require the parish nurse to offer the patient other alternatives for care. As a health educator, the parish nurse will provide information about diseases and treatments and encourage the patient to ask questions about treatment and medications. These nursing functions that encourage patient independence may be viewed as interfering with the practice of medicine and create areas of conflict.

Empowerer

A key function of the parish nurse is to empower people to take charge of their own health. She can do this in a myriad of ways. Perhaps the most important is to serve as a resource about the health care services available in the community, from twelve-step programs to complementary health care practitioners, nutritionists, and medical specialists. By networking with other health care providers in the community (to locate free mammogram services and other preventive treatments), the parish nurse can open doors for people who then will be able to take healing into their own hands.

The parish nurse serves as a liaison between the church and a variety of community resources and services and often advocates on behalf of parishioners with these agencies. The complexity of the current health care system may overwhelm the average person, and parish nurses can help keep their parishioners from getting lost in the system. Parishioners have reported that they are tremendously grateful to the parish nurses for introducing them to many types of care they did not know existed. This may be especially true for those who are suffering from addictions and need self-help and support groups as well as information about treatment facilities; victims of domestic violence who are afraid to talk to anyone else can unburden themselves to the parish nurse.

Empowerment to heal by serving as a resource can take many forms. One parish nurse was asked to conduct a vigil service for a baby in her church who had died from SIDS (sudden infant death syndrome). The parish nurse prepared her sermon by calling the national hot line to find out all the medical facts about SIDS. By sharing information about SIDS during the vigil service, she communicated to family and friends that no one had neglected the baby. She conveyed to the parents that it was not their fault that their baby had died and they should not blame themselves. The parish nurse empowered the parents to be healed by supplying them with the medical facts to release them from their own sense of culpability. Hearing the facts from a nurse provided the parents with confidence in the information they could not have obtained from a preacher. This combination of the scientific with the spiritual and psychological was a healing moment for the family.

Health Educator

The parish nurse can fulfill the function of prevention by being a health educator. The nurse teaches or uses others to lead courses, seminars, and workshops for the congregation on a wide variety of health-related topics such as health maintenance, disease prevention, early detection through screening, the role of emotions in illness and, most important, an introduction to the interrelation of body and soul.

Through a variety of formats—seminars, conferences, classes, workshops, small discussion groups, individual sessions, newsletters, printed educational materials, and bulletin boards—the parish nurse seeks to raise the health awareness of the parish community and to foster an understanding of the relationship between lifestyle, personal habits, attitudes, faith, and well-being. She can offer workshops on a wide range of bioethical dilemmas and other health-related topics.

The nurse supplements her teaching with programs that feature qualified speakers from medicine, public health, physical therapy, social work, nutrition, and psychology, as well as ethics and theology. Physicians from the congregation also speak on their own specialties or general health concerns.

The nurse organizes and finds facilitators (possibly herself) for groups centered on particular issues such as weight loss, diabetes, divorce, stress management, arthritis, youth problems, problems of loss and grief, children of aging parents, and so forth.

Through health education, a parish nurse may highlight a monthly theme that conforms to the theme being promoted by the local health department or the American Medical Association. For example, a theme on the healthy heart prompted a man in a congregation who knew CPR (cardiopulmonary resuscitation) to come forward and volunteer to give free CPR classes to church members. Another monthly theme on nutrition inspired a long-time parishioner who had recently lost seventy-eight pounds to share his joy and regime with other church members struggling with their weight. The individual formed a Weight Watchers group and called it "Soul Weights" (as a takeoff on Soul Mates), which now meets every two weeks at the church. Some people weigh in; others do not. Some have formed a walking group. About fourteen church members attend.

Of course, not every educational attempt is a success. Even though the parish nurse got an oncology nurse to launch a breast cancer awareness month one Sunday at her church, no one came. At another church, some church members walked out of a video presentation on how to do self-breast examinations because they were troubled by what they perceived as immodesty.

Often a parish nurse can spot a misdiagnosis. An active church member who complained of insomnia had been prescribed Benadryl by a doctor. Encountering the individual at church, the parish nurse first prayed with the man and then talked to him as they sat on a pew at the back of the church. The man soon disclosed his problems: he was sending money to his son who was in a drug rehabilitation center; he did not know what to do, and the problem was keeping him up at night. It was disturbing him so much, he was drinking heavily. Then the man revealed he was an alcoholic. His wife had been asking him to stop drinking for some time, but he could not see his wife's point of view. He needed another view. By listening to the man, the parish nurse helped him see his problem from another perspective, after which he started attending Alcoholics Anonymous.

Grief support groups are another avenue parish nurses use to help prevent disease and addictive and destructive behavior. Grief support groups are essential for children and adults going though divorce, death in the family, or a change of job to take them through the stages of grief and relieve the stress that results in disease. Grief support groups are invaluable to help immigrants name their unclaimed sorrow that stems from the pain of immigration, the confusion of a new language and who they are in a new land. The lack of support in this area explains why so many immigrant adolescents are in gangs and involved in drugs.

Trainer

One of the parish nurse's functions is to find volunteers who are naturally warm, understanding, and willing to listen to hurting people. These volunteers can be instructed to do even better what they are already doing naturally. They can become additional hands, ears, and eyes for the nurse as they make house calls on the sick, serve as small group study leaders, and participate in many other tasks. In large congregations the nurse by herself cannot begin to respond to all the needs, so trained volunteers can add tremendously to her effectiveness.

The parish nurse may guide volunteers to reach out, for example, to individuals who have recently sustained a loss or to families attempting to care for a family member recently discharged from the hospital. The services needed and provided are as varied as the human needs encountered.[17]

This training function is distinguished from the empowering one because the nurse is training church volunteers to be health workers with members of the congregation. The parish nurse's training function is central to home visitation programs that many churches have successfully launched with a cadre of volunteers under the direction of a volunteer leader, who in turn is trained by the parish nurse. The parish nurse at one church, for example, holds potlucks twice a year for the leader and twenty-two volunteers of her home visitation program. There, the volunteers are trained on how to listen effectively, start conversations, and pray with the people they visit. More technical training is required for the volunteers who agree to help the parish nurse with blood pressure screenings and inoculations. Often, the parish nurse trains pastoral staff in health education so they can minister more effectively to congregants. A priest asked the parish nurse, for example, to explain to him why babies are stillborn so that he could better counsel a family who was grieving in this situation. (One might wonder if he should have simply sent the parish nurse to meet with them.)

Personal Health Counselor

Creating an atmosphere in which parishioners are comfortable in sharing concerns, the parish nurse is available to all parishioners to discuss personal health problems, to recommend medical intervention when necessary, and to make home, hospital, and nursing home visits. This may be especially important in a medical emergency when family members are out of town.

The parish nurse usually works with members of the congregation, but also works with some nonmembers. She fills a missing ingredient in the health care system by providing a professional listening ear, assessing health problems, recommending and/or providing minor health care measures, and making referrals to physicians and/or community support services. She educates individuals in specific ways that they might better care for themselves and communicates good health concepts as a role model. She may also help people with instructions about their medications.

Minor health problems, when detected early, can be prevented from developing later into major illnesses. Likewise, individuals may be unaware of the relationship between their lifestyle and personal habits and their health problems. The visibility and availability of a parish nurse help parishioners recognize, acknowledge, and seek treatment for symptoms they might otherwise have ignored or denied. Also, the presence of the parish nurse may encourage parishioners to take more responsibility for their own health.

Often church members will approach the parish nurse with a physical ailment only to confess spiritual or psychological problems. At one parish in San Jose, California, an elderly woman came for a blood pressure screening. Her reading was alarmingly high, and the parish nurse suggested she see a doctor nearby. The woman said she had no problems, and the parish nurse invited her for lunch. It was over lunch that the woman opened up and told a story of benign neglect. She had recently arrived in the United States from Peru to be with her youngest son and his family, but they considered her meddlesome and said they did not want her to be so involved in their lives. The elderly woman was distraught. The parish nurse listened to the woman tell her story for five hours and then took her blood pressure; it was back to normal. The parish nurse counseled the woman to return to her homeland to be with her eldest son; there she would be happier, well cared for in a culture that honors the elderly.

Spiritual Counselor

This function is not to be a counselor in the technical sense of the word but to assist people to explore matters of health and faith. Unaddressed grief is believed to be one of the primary causes of people's mental and physical diseases, and it often manifests itself in anger. Parish nurses can help address this by encouraging people to cry and not to hold back their tears at funerals. One parish nurse considers her work with grieving families at funerals to be central to her health ministry. At the vigil service the night before a funeral, she helps the family plan the funeral and makes sure that each member of the family has a role to play in the service.

The parish nurse may assist overwrought people to decide what they should do and how to work with the pastor/priest/rabbi to plan the service. At a Catholic church in California, there had been a suicide/murder in which the husband had poured gasoline on himself and his wife and lit the flames that killed them as their two children, ages six and eight, watched. The parish nurse saw the children being excluded from the funeral planning process. She saw the critical need for them to be involved so they could find an outlet for their trauma. She adapted the existing liturgy to more fully incorporate and respond to the family needs. The children sprinkled the holy water on the coffins of their parents and took the flowers off their parents' coffins in order for the pall to be placed on the father's coffin by his brother and on the mother's coffin by her two sisters. These small acts made a great difference to the grieving children.

Some parish nurses are directly linked to the worship service by being trained to be chalice bearers at communion. Quite a few churches have healing stations where the parish nurse and trained volunteers stand on communion Sundays, either to the side of the pulpit or at the back of the church in the narthex, to hear the concerns of the people and pray for them while anointing them with consecrated oil in the name of Christ.

One parish nurse, Jean Wright-Elson, tells of the woman who said to her, "I wish to be healed of my breast lump." Alarmed that the woman might think prayer alone would address her problem, the nurse whispered that the woman should see her after the service. The woman did, and the parish nurse counseled her to see a doctor, which the woman had been avoiding because of her fear of the medical establishment. Through more prayer and the assurance that the parish nurse would accompany her to the doctor, the woman went to the hospital and discovered the lump was malignant and needed to be treated with chemotherapy. A radical mastectomy was not necessary because the lump was detected at the early stages.

Provider of Health Services

Within the limits of nursing education and licenses, parish nurses can provide some health services. Blood pressure screenings are very popular because they are noninvasive. They are also highly effective tools in preventive medicine; the three top killers—strokes, heart attacks, and diabetes—can be detected with a blood pressure reading. Churches are ideal locations for flu and other inoculations.

Some parish nurses have medical equipment for loan such as walkers, wheelchairs, crutches, commodes, and beds. The borrowers sign a liability form stating that they are borrowing the equipment from the church as a service to parishioners, and they will not sue the church if it does not work. In one church, the request for equipment was so great that the parish nurse said the place looked like Lourdes.

A related ministry may spring from direct services. In visiting a church member who had diabetes, for example, a parish nurse discovered the man had to stand on the corner and jump in a truck to get work as a migrant worker—work for which he often was not paid or which resulted in abuse. The parish nurse wrote a grant and received $200,000 to start a job center for migrant workers where they could find one of the few public showers in the city and decent work at a fair wage. General concern with welfare reform has led other churches to band together to combine resources in order to feed the poor.

Some churches have care teams that parish nurses organize and coordinate to respond to people who have been hospitalized and then are homebound upon release. One group of volunteers on the care team prepares food for a week to take to the patient; another group focuses on providing volunteers to pray with the individual on a daily basis; still another group helps around the house and gardens; if she can, the parish nurse tries to find someone who has suffered the same ailment in order to encourage the patient.

THE FUTURE OF PARISH NURSING

Parish nursing is developing so rapidly that future projections are hard to chart. As more parish nurses become incorporated into the health care system, they may become bureaucratized with reports and forms. If this serendipitous response to health needs becomes overly institutionalized, the unique contribution of parish nursing may be lost.

Joni Goodnight, a former president of Health Ministries Association, wrote, "Most of us in parish nursing love it because we're able to speak about Christ. We're encouraged to pray with our clients, and we're rewarded by seeing the peace that envelops them when they feel God's spiritual healing in their lives."[18] Parish nursing has become the ideal way of bringing together professional skills and one's faith. If parish nurses become public health nurses, they will have lost a valuable opportunity to change the face of health care in this country—not simply health education with a spiritual overlay.

Another challenge facing parish nursing is whether it can become truly interfaith. Although the movement has been ecumenical from the outset, it has been strongest in Lutheran, Presbyterian, Methodist, and Roman Catholic parishes. By the late 1990s, some Jewish congregations hired parish nurses, and those from Eastern religions are exploring this model. The question is whether the raison d'être of this specialty will lose its uniqueness and theological dimension in seeking the lowest common religious denominator or be enriched by those of different faiths.

9

Starting a Health Ministry

Although parish nurses, as discussed in the last chapter, are often instrumental in starting a health ministry, this chapter suggests specific ways that a church or group of churches can start a health ministry. This use of the word is referring not to the discipline but to the approach and programs.

"If Jesus came to bring life and to bring it abundantly, Christians cannot stand by and watch their neighbors suffer without trying to do something. To start a ministry, you begin! The compassion of Christ is the motivating force."[1] The pastor may be the one who needs to raise the awareness of the congregation concerning the need for a health ministry, but it is important at the start to engage the church members. Planning together, recruiting and training volunteers, raising the necessary money, and setting realistic goals at a time frame that will facilitate success are crucial. The pastor will serve in numerous ways but, most important, will build coalitions with government agencies and community groups. She needs vision and persistence.[2]

Denis Duncan, a British theologian, discusses ways to set up a healing ministry program and suggests several priorities: (1) to create a group whose weekly purpose is to intercede for people in need; (2) to set up a Bible study group whose purpose is to reflect on matters of faith and healing; and (3) to preach and teach on the role of the church.[3] The emphasis here is on the involvement of the whole church so that the ministry is not viewed as a special sidelight of either a fringe group or a so-called more spiritual group.

THE STEPS TO FORM A HEALTH MINISTRY

Many of the steps to forming a health ministry that are outlined here are to be done concurrently. When one is learning about health ministries and researching community needs, praying for guidance and doing Bible study are vital. The ministry should begin modestly and expand on existing resources, both people and money. The steps described here are offered to give as much information on the subject as possible. No need to digest or follow it all; simply take it; use what is helpful. There is no set formula. Health ministries programs are truly the work of the Holy Spirit and take on a life of their own depending upon each individual situation. No two ministries will be alike—nor should they be.

Become Knowledgeable about Health Ministry

The first step in starting a health ministry is to recognize that it should never be a solo enterprise.[4] Even in the information-gathering phase, partnering with other people enriches the ministry. A small group of people who share an interest in health ministries may work together. People in congregations may actually be practicing health ministries without realizing it. For example, Meals on Wheels, nursery schools, homebound visitation, and prayer circles are part of a health ministry. Learn how others' programs began and what the obstacles and keys to success were in establishing them.

Many denominations have a centralized health ministries office or programs from which to obtain information and resources. Community resources can also be excellent information sources. Local hospitals and medical centers often offer support groups and health education classes. The local twelve-step programs, for example, or nearby wholistic health care centers may become potential partners for a health ministry. Using consultants may help think through the important issues.

Use Available Resource Organizations. Resource organizations establish membership or networks both nationally and internationally to research and formulate policy or opinion and disseminate information on health care issues. These groups provide a public arena for denominational or interdenominational discussion. They may provide information that is used by churches or groups in establishing their own health ministries. Ideally, resource organizations help congregations avoid duplication of effort in establishing health care ministries by centralizing information pertinent to specific ministries.

They provide ways of educating church members and the community at large about the importance of the church as a provider and resource of health care instead of churches having to invent programs from scratch. A local congregation can function as a resource organization by offering health care information to its members and the community.

Resource organizations may be established at the denominational level to centralize information on health ministries for member churches; or they may provide ecumenical resources through newsletters, conferences, and special publications. They may be agencies of the church, parachurch groups, or academic research or community-based organizations, which identify potential constituents as church members. These groups provide a public arena for denominational or interdenominational discussion and may frequently take a public stance on particular issues, for example, reproductive options, physician-assisted suicide, or health care information. They may also sponsor workshops, conferences, seminars, and conferences for their constituents.[5]

Clarify the Definition of Health Ministry

Either the pastor or a lay leader can clarify what is meant by health ministry and what programs are needed in a particular area. Before beginning a health ministry, its mission must be clear.

Establishing one's own perspective is accomplished by reflecting upon health ministry material, listening to the needs of one's immediate community, and praying. Each setting requires different styles to address the situation. Adapting general information about health ministries to one's own situation through personal reflection is helpful. Defining health ministry in relation to a specific context is the starting point. Perhaps in the process of "recapturing the vision of the church" one's own self-understanding as a minister or a lay leader will also change.

One of the necessary decisions is whether to adopt a broad or narrow focus in health ministries. Some groups, for example, the Institute for Development Training, have chosen women's health and specifically reproductive choice and family planning and operate in one specific area of health ministries. Others such as National Capital Presbytery Health Ministries followed a very comprehensive agenda working on AIDS, disabilities, elderly needs, and drug abuse; they saw their mission as multifaceted.

Both the laity and the clergy of a congregation should be involved in determining the course of the health ministry. They need each other. Cecil Williams, pastor at Glide Memorial Church in San Francisco, California, observed of his attempt to solve other people's problems, "In so doing, I short-circuited their power and tried to play God. I exhausted myself and lost myself trying to protect people from claiming the responsibility for their own lives. That delusion of being a healer allowed me to put all of my energy into someone else. There had to be a way to care for myself while still being an agent for change in the community."6 Williams found his personal calling in liberation theology—empowering others.

People may challenge whether the church should even be involved in health ministries; some people believe that the church's role as a healer ended with the apostles. Part of starting a health ministry is having a vision of health as a wholistic integration of body, mind, and spirit.7

The biblical concept of *shalom* speaks of wholeness and wellness, of the total well-being of individuals and communities. It arises out of a covenant relationship characterized by love toward God (one of the parties of the covenant) and love to neighbor and self (the other party in the covenant). When these qualities characterize the lives of individuals and communities, there is health in the person and in the community. There is *shalom*.8

The definition of health as wholeness and sickness as brokenness forces us to see the whole person in his or her setting. Healing then includes a wide variety of activities and factors that move us toward wholeness, especially religious values and spiritual resources. The biblical perspective emphasizes the community dimension of healing, which is caring for the ill person in his or her milieu.

Understand the Role of the Pastor

As ministers of healing, pastors are in need of healing. By starting with their own understanding of health, they can set an example of a healthy lifestyle for members of their congregation and the community. By refusing to be slaves to society's addiction to overwork and materialism, they can offer a healthy alternative. Pastors can assist people in rethinking ways of living that can bring wholistic health. Part of understanding health ministry is seeing the pastor himself or herself as part of the health ministry.

Consider that as one who ministers in Christ's name, the pastor is a healer in several ways. First, the pastor proclaims universal truths: each person has infinite worth; illness is not necessarily a sign of sin; when sin does cause illness, forgiveness is available; death, though our enemy, has been conquered and no longer needs to be feared. Pointing to God's love as reflected in all healing is crucial and may include showing how all diagnosis, prognosis, and therapy involves christological dimensions.

Second, the pastor conveys the symbols of health and healing, relating to people as persons, not patients. As people face sickness and struggle to accept and overcome the undeniable fact of their own fragility, symbols of healing may involve sustenance in the face of pain and suffering—assisting people to live in the midst of their brokenness.

Third, the pastor counsels individuals in order to reveal spiritual road-blocks to healing; put people in touch with their own inner resources for healing; open them to God's power of healing; and integrate them into a support and service community. Trustworthiness and constancy are part of the counseling ministry.[9]

Form a Health Ministry Committee

As discussed earlier, starting a health ministry should not be a solo enterprise. It is imperative to form a committee, that is, a health cabinet, immediately so that this program is a communal endeavor. The pastor may function as a chief of staff to which the cabinet reports. In any case, the committee should always be approved by the pastor. An associate health minister and/or parish nurse may be appointed to head the cabinet, who reports to the pastor. However, the Health Ministries Association recommends selecting a chairperson other than the health minister or parish nurse to direct the health ministry, develop goals, and provide support, assistance, guidance, and evaluation for the health minister or parish nurse.[10]

While the pastor and health minister and/or parish nurse are key members of the health cabinet, church members who are interested in health issues are also ideal candidates. These people are not necessarily health professionals (though this would be advantageous), but they should have an affinity for a wholistic approach to health involving mind, body, and spirit, and be attuned to their own health. The health cabinet and the pastor should meet regularly to pray, read, and brainstorm together. There should be ongoing education and support for those in this ministry.[11]

It is essential to include members from a variety of interest groups within the congregation, those who are involved with youth, women's and men's ministries, the elderly, and outreach ministries. A core group of leaders who are representative of the congregation will ensure a sense of ownership and commitment to the programs.

It may be important for the cabinet to have reading materials and books on the subject if they are unfamiliar with it. The Christian vocation and spirituality project of Suzanne Farnham was initiated by a group of leaders reading the major classical texts on spiritual formation to stimulate their own thinking. This eventually led to a new form of discernment and spiritual direction combining Ignatian and Quaker spirituality.[12]

The Health Ministries Association, in its detailed *"How to" Manual*, recommends that the cabinet specifically should be responsible for the following:

- Evaluation of the most appropriate organizational position for the health committee.
- Establishment of purpose and goals.
- Identification of resources within the congregation, such as volunteers, health professionals, educators, funders, administrators.
- Identification of resources in the community in order to avoid duplication.
- Determination of which health-care model to pursue.
- Development of the budget and fund raising plan.
- Recruitment and hiring of the health minister and/or parish nurse.[13]

Pray for God's Direction

To determine its ministry, a congregation should pray for guidance to discern the needs and best use of the gifts of the congregation. Bishop Morris Maddocks counsels us to become a praying church. Church leaders are responsible to encourage and enable the use of God's gifts to us, so "that the Church may truly become the Church." When people know how to pray together, they come to know God "in the context of the Christian family."[14] Decide what type of prayer seems to work best for a particular congregation: public prayers of the people during worship services; prayer groups or healing teams; or a combination of some or all of these. Expect the Holy Spirit to work amazing things as one is open to God's leading.[15]

The more groups there are, Maddocks says, praying and being involved in community activities, the sounder will be the structure.[16] For example, at the heart of the health ministry in Kingston, Jamaica, are prayer teams in the church who are willing to "exercise their faith in a ministry of healing." They pray "regularly for sick members of the church and community; invite ill persons to meet with the group for special prayer; have a visitation program for the sick; and pray before services for God's blessing."[17]

The aim of the Guild of St. Raphael in the United Kingdom, for example, is prayer ministry "to promote the belief that God wills the conquest of disease" and to guide people to the knowledge that "Christ is the source of all healing." The sick are taught to recognize the need for repentance and faith; to use the Eucharist, anointing, and laying on of hands for healing; to pray and use meditation.[18]

Educate Your Congregation

Bible Study. Health ministry cabinet members and the congregation at large should be encouraged to attend Bible study sessions that foster reflection on Christ's healing ministry and how it relates to the local community. Much of the material in my companion volume can be used as the basis for Bible study and adult education programs.

D. S. Allister's *Sickness and Healing in the Church* contains scriptural passages for use in sessions on this subject.[19] Carl Geores recommends following a five-step Bible study process as the cornerstone in establishing any community development and health ministry model:

1. The Great Commission—Evangelism (Matthew 28:16–20)
2. Connecting the Gospel to the World (Luke 4:16–20)
3. Servant Church (John 13:1–17; Mark 10:36–45)
4. Connecting to One Another—Cooperation (I Corinthians 12:12–31)
5. Equipping Members for Ministry (Ephesians 4:11–16)[20]

Preaching. The pastor should preach about the "connection between spirituality and health."[21] Sermons should take into consideration "healthy lifestyles involving choices about whether or not to smoke or drink; how much exercise to get; whether to eat a nourishing diet; how to handle anger; how to handle stress; how to nourish the spiritual aspects of our life."[22] The healing aspects of the regular worship services can be emphasized and sound theology expounded.

Informal Conversation. One of the most effective ways to educate the congregation about health ministry is to talk with the members. Listen to the members' concerns about their health and what they perceive to be the stresses in their lives. Share with them how the church can help, and recruit them to become involved in some aspect of health ministry.

A health ministry is not accomplished by pulpit announcements or notices. It happens through person-to-person contact while praying for God's guidance; getting to know the needs of people in the congregation is crucial.[23]

Retreats. A two-day health awareness retreat involving easy travel and an overnight stay can be an ideal setting for educating people about health ministries. The retreat can include worship services that touch the brokenness of people and point to healing as well as small group interaction to gain insight into the physical, emotional, spiritual, or social factors causing health concerns, with a commitment to solve them. I led several such intergenerational church retreats in Washington, D.C., where information and activities were geared to different groups within the churches. These retreats can focus families on health and provide deep reflection for all ages.

Dissemination of Information. Church bulletins, newsletters, bulletin boards, and literature tables are logical places to share information. Presentations on health ministries to groups and committees in the church are important. Creating a health ministry section in the church library can be an easy way of making information available.[24]

Lay Health Advisors. Educating the congregation can be assisted by developing a special group called lay health advisors. These advisors offer eight weeks of training in common health issues, the church's biblical and historical calling to care for the poor and sick, and ways to care for the whole person—both body and spirit. "Lay leaders promote wellness and healthier lifestyles in their church congregations, monitor those who are chronically ill, and identify those who may be developing serious illnesses."[25]

One of the most important areas of lay ministry is that of intercessory prayer. A listening ministry and visitation are significant. Listening ministries offer the unhurried and uncritical ear to people who otherwise are bypassed by doctors, nurses, health visitors, and clergy because of their busy schedules. These are examples of health ministries that do not have monetary costs but involve volunteer time.[26]

Continuing Education. Using health care professionals as seminar leaders is an ideal way to continue health education in your congregation. Outside consultants can be brought in to speak about particular health concerns in an adult education series. Continuing education should be a primary component of the parish nurse's service to the congregation. The programs described in the next chapter offer further ideas for keeping interest in health ministries alive.

Assess Church and Community Needs

It is wise to begin a health ministry by identifying needs within the church so that the members can see a direct impact on their lives. Many successful programs begin by meeting the needs of one individual or family. The corollary is to "identify resources within the congregation—volunteers, health professionals, educators, administrators," or corporation executives—whose interest is in meeting these needs. Also assess community resources and programs "to avoid duplication" of efforts. "Find out where resources are inadequate, inaccessible or unavailable."[27] Focus on what the congregation does best.

A congregation may overlook the resource of its own facility to offer to the community. Providing space for group meetings for such organizations as twelve-step addiction recovery programs is an obvious ministry because every parish includes people who suffer from addictions. People from the community can become part of a weekly Bible study group to help the congregation discern the mission and function of the health ministry.

The church should help the community identify its problems and develop the solutions. People should define their needs, not let someone else define them.[28] Empowering the community to deal with the problems that have caused their need is much more effective in the long term than simply giving them a solution. People need to be involved in solving their own problems. The needs of a rural Baptist church may be different from those of a suburban Presbyterian one.

Using one's imagination in tackling a problem in the community is central. Traditional solutions do not suit every community, as the culture, the history of relationships and the way of interacting with each other influences the ministry's solutions. Rather than having your community think the problem rests with them rather than the cure, try changing the cure.[29]

One health ministry, established in an impoverished area, linked art and health including storytelling, art and sculpture workshops, and dance and movement for overweight people (Bromley by Bow Centre). Another ministry in Saint Marylebone Parish in London (the former Churches Council for Health and Healing) found space for a health ministry by clearing away the large number of coffins in its extensive crypt, reburying them in a nearby cemetery, and using the vacated space for the living instead of the dead. Besides a counseling ministry and medical practice, this ministry offered a music therapy unit where a team of music therapists who were Christians helpd people achieve a greater degree of wholeness through sound. These projects illustrate that defining a health ministry depends on the available resources and the nature of the community.

In starting a primary health care service, working with the local hospitals to get their support will deflect potential competitive difficulties. One church congregation that was providing health care to the poor was sued by several private medical practitioners in the neighborhood for unfair competition. Though the church had gained support from the large, local hospital, it had failed to establish productive relationships with the individual practitioners in the area.

Identify Existing Health Ministries Programs

Recognize that the ongoing ministries of worship, such as the sacraments, and pastoral counseling already qualify as health ministries. If a church is hosting Alcoholics Anonymous or other twelve-step meetings, or participating in Meals-on-Wheels programs, these are health ministries programs. Health ministries are already functioning even if they are not named as such. The areas for a church-based health ministry elaborated in chapter 3 may help identify existing health ministries.

Determine the Nature and Type of Your Ministries

Partnerships—Central for an Effective Health Ministries Program. Network with hospitals, health departments, and other community organizations to provide a solid base for the health ministry. A health ministry may involve a single church or work jointly with other local congregations to tackle a community need. This is an especially shrewd strategy for smaller congregations that do not have the resources to have their own health cabinet. By pooling resources, churches can form a powerful coalition, gaining the political voice to find the funds they need. Many successful health ministries have been started this way to fight drug addiction or to offer direct health services to the community.[30]

Choosing your partners in health ministry can determine its success and longevity. For example, one church-based antidrug campaign was involved significantly with law enforcement personnel. The campaign was successful in eliminating drugs from the neighborhood community through vigilant efforts by volunteer members of the church who provided information to the police. However, the question remains whether a church wants to be so closely identified with law enforcement: Does the short-term success merit the church's alignment with one sector of the community, that is, law enforcement and the establishment, perhaps shutting out marginalized community members?

Congregational, Community Outreach, or Both. Will the health ministry serve only congregation members, or will it focus on community need? Of course, the two may overlap. Generally, it is better to begin with congregational needs, but also to assess the neighborhood. Vital, alive churches, according to Donald Smith, who studies such congregations, look outside their immediate congregation; they grow as they practice real mission. Many of the health ministries programs described in the next chapter followed that model.[31]

Solo Congregation or Collaboratively with Other Churches. Large congregations can often do a solo health ministry. A small congregation with limited resources may want to join hands with a cluster of small churches in the region—either from the same denomination or from different denominations. Forming a church cluster does not happen quickly, advises Carl Geores, who developed a highly effective cluster-church approach in Leeds,

Maine, over a period of many years (Ministry in the North Country [MINC]). It is the result of a teaching ministry that includes preaching, adult Bible study, community needs evaluation, and mission design development; a systematic approach is needed.

A compassionate, pastoral ministry should extend to the larger community, encouraging the congregation to develop a concern for all people. When a congregation uncovers the needs in the community, it will also become aware of the importance of partners and joining in a cooperative ministry with neighboring congregations. The Leeds community ministry style can be applicable to health ministries.

Begin by identifying interested churches and studying the community needs. Representatives need to be chosen from congregations who carry authority and can speak for the church. They can share their own ministries, and the group can determine what joint ministries are possible. Once the programs are chosen, then a mission design with goals and objectives and a review process needs to be decided. A fund-raising plan is crucial, as is the establishment of the governing body, its authority and mission, method of choosing representatives, number of officers, responsibilities, terms of office, and job descriptions. If the project is large in scope, such as establishing a wholistic health care center, incorporation may be necessary.

Religious Affiliation. Deciding if the ministry will be interfaith, ecumenical, or single denomination will radically affect its mission. Many leaders believe that health ministry is ideally suited to be interfaith because of the common understanding concerning the link between spirituality and health, whether Buddhist, Muslim, Jewish, Christian, or Hindu. "Spirituality is the unifying and integrative aspect of a person's life and when lived intentionally, is experienced as a process of growth and maturity."[32]

Our spiritual heritage is the basis for community and participation in meeting shared needs. Though the content of spirituality will differ among various faith traditions, there can be mutual respect and an openness to learn from one another. This involves commitment to one another to give full expression to our faith rather than seeking the least common denominator, in worship as well as dialogue. Our "highest common denominator" is the importance of spirituality for health, unifying us for health promotion. The most successful interfaith ministries are "centered around a common activity or purpose (food giving, caregiving, social ministry); common faith concerns (interfaith dialogue); and common prayer to God (interfaith worship)." The advantage of interfaith ministries is that we are stronger together than apart. The disadvantage is that a removal of boundaries threatens one's sense of security, and the faith basis for the activity may be minimized.[33]

Implicitly or Explicitly Christian. Related to the questions about whether a health ministry should be ecumenical or interfaith is whether the health ministry will be implicitly or explicitly Christian. Some health ministries are implicitly Christian in their theology, staff members, and funding. However, externally they may not look like a Christian organization. There are no Bibles, prayer books, theological literature, or crosses in their health centers, nor do their brochures or posters explain their theological roots. Eschewing overt Christian symbols, they take instead an implicit, central paradigm of the broken and resurrected Christ who meets people in their weakness and uses their weakness as a means of salvation. What emerges is a ministry of caring whose motivation and roots are Christian but not overtly so.

For these groups their decision to underplay their Christian roots is intentional in order to identify the health ministry with the community rather than the institutional church. They may adopt a prophetic role, which calls into question all institutions. The former Ombersley Road Surgery, now called the Balsam Heath Practice in Birmingham, England, is one such example.

Health ministries programs must not become Christianized versions of secular community programs with no marked difference. Unfortunately, that happened to both the educational institutions and the hospitals that were founded by the church in the nineteenth century. Most of them have gradually become indistinguishable from state-run institutions, and many of them were turned over to the state. For example, the Roman Catholic hospitals system's biggest threat is whether they will become for-profit hospitals, losing much of their raison d'être to treat patients independently of their ability to pay.

However, a tension needs to be maintained here. Sometimes it is time to let go and let the ministry flow back into the secular world. The question is: Will it maintain its effectiveness if it loses its connection with the healing source of Christ?

The Staff. Naturally, the selection of staff for the health ministries will be influenced by the type of program; volunteers should also be considered staff. In other words, the staffing decision should take a comprehensive look at the total work to be done by both paid and volunteer staff. The advantage of volunteers is their sense of ownership and their ability to begin immediately. The disadvantage is their limited time and the unevenness of their commitment and abilities. The size of the church and the nature of the health ministry programs will determine the number and type of staff positions. Many new health ministries have turned to the parish nurse as the person to start health ministries. Although there are many, many pluses to having a parish nurse or health minister, it may not be the panacea we think.

However, parish nurses may be "naturals" to promote health care in the congregation because they focus on preventive help—before people become sick. They also care for people within the community of faith, offering the added spiritual dimension that could tip the balance in favor of motivating parishioners to change an unhealthy lifestyle. That is perhaps why these parish nurses are often referred to as "ministers of health."

The health cabinet can recruit and hire the health minister and/or parish nurse, and write a job description for each position. The parish nurse would more specifically address preventive health care through education of the congregation, while the health minister's focus would be broader based with less medical expertise and more organizational and community outreach activities. However, the parish nurse could function as the health minister.

Develop a Financial Plan

Financing new programs can appear daunting at first. Because many small churches believe they do not have the resources either of people or of money to do programs, they must plan carefully. Many an outstanding program has ended due to the lack of sound financial planning. The first step is to begin a new program modestly, creating a budget that includes dollars and in-kind services. This will prove helpful in seeking foundation funding, if necessary; matching funding of local support and an ongoing financial base are crucial criteria for receiving outside grants. Money follows ideas. Sharing a vision of what a particular health ministry can accomplish attracts funds. People like to see concretely how their money is making a difference; if clear needs are recognized and practical programs are created to meet these needs, the money will follow.

In terms of the modest beginnings mentioned earlier, realistically assessing the people and monetary resources available is central to ensure long-term success. Launching a new program, for example, a ministry with persons with AIDS and their families, in a church that is judgmental and afraid of AIDS will create funding difficulties. If several needs are identified, it is best to select one visible need, for example, respite care for caregivers of aging persons, which makes the initial fund-raising easier. When those program moneys are secured, one can move to more controversial programs. (This strategy is not always advocated; sometimes entering into unpopular and controversial areas may be where our faith calls us even in light of the financial uncertainty.)

Any health ministries committee needs to have at least one person who is an expert in finances both for planning and for accounting purposes. Overexpenditures and under-budget income items can cause a program to fail even if it is important and worthwhile. In addition to developing a budget and raising money, creative financing is important. For congregations that have access to funding, the Health Ministries Association's "*How to" Manual* identifies some common financial arrangements.[34]

Respond to New Needs

A church may launch a ministry whose success causes it to be embraced by the community. At that point, one may need to let go and allow the Holy Spirit to continue to guide the effort. A key function of health ministry as an enabling body may be to work itself out of a job in order to empower the local community.

In addition, the ministry may need to change to respond to new needs. One highly successful health ministry realized its practice would become irrelevant if it refused to grow and change with its population (the Balsam Health Practice). Its constituency originally were marginalized immigrants who after ten years were entering into the mainstream of British society in Birmingham, England, so needed a different type of health care practice.

A CAVEAT

My experience of founding and directing a health ministries program for nearly a decade in Washington, D.C., gave me some insights into the ingredients for an effective health ministries program. The National Capital Presbytery Health Ministries existed from 1983 to 1993. Many of its programs were assumed by local churches, but it might have continued as an entity if certain guidelines had been followed. (Of course, it should also be noted that at that time health ministry was a fledgling concept.) First, having direct service programs with visible results is important for a program to gain the necessary support. Second, a health ministries board needs experts in fund-raising so this is not the sole responsibility of the director. Third, training your successor beforehand so that the program is not overly dependent on one person's expertise is crucial. Many health ministries start with great hope but become too dependent on a single visionary leader. When that leader leaves, the program collapses. Fourth, create programs that are self-supporting and not dependent for their continuance on outside funding.

The Health Ministries Association cites several other factors that facilitate success in a congregational health ministry:

- Involve congregational members from the beginning.
- Assess needs/wants through a survey of congregation members.
- Publicize information from the survey to the membership and let the health committee use it when planning health ministry programs.
- Prioritize the needs; begin slowly.
- Meet regularly as a health committee with the pastor to apprise him or her of plans, goals, and membership needs.
- Provide "ongoing education and support for those engaged in the ministry," especially for volunteers.[35]

10

Practical Programs
for Healthy People

N ow that we have reviewed the history of the church's healing ministry and the wonderful opportunity for the church to redefine and expand its health ministry, I will describe effective programs that, I hope, will inspire and energize us to become involved in a healing ministry.

PROGRAM SELECTION CRITERIA

In the late 1970s and early 1980s the term "health ministries" was seldom, if ever, used for the church's involvement in healing ministries; now some describe this as a new discipline. In fact, National Capital Presbytery Health Ministries, established in 1983, may have been one of the first so named. It published a directory of health ministries consisting of forty-six programs principally concentrated in metropolitan Washington, D.C. The selection of the ones to include was relatively straightforward because there were fewer than one hundred in the United States at that time.[1] In the late 1990s the task is more daunting since they have expanded to thousands.

The programs included here were selected to be representative of geographic diversity—urban, rural, suburban—throughout the United States and a few international programs; style of ministry—solo congregation, coalition of churches, ecumenical, and interfaith; sponsorship—health care institutions, community agencies, corporations, denominational headquarters, local congregations; cross-cultural and racial/ethnic diversity; and different categories—educational, support/advocacy, and direct health care services. (Several of these groups work in two or more categories but are listed in the category of their primary activity.)

"Health ministry" is defined as any program that meets a broad base of health-related needs and is founded and supported by or related to a church or religious group or body. Groups that were contacted self-determined if they fit this definition. In addition, the longevity of the ministry was an important criterion for inclusion. Many programs are short-lived as their charismatic founders move on to other endeavors.

To achieve uniform information, a computerized data-gathering instrument was developed with thirty-nine questions requiring short, quantifiable answers about budget, staff, governance, type of program, and so forth. Most of the programs described here have been visited by either the author or her assistant, Jane Ferguson. Their descriptions were reviewed by the program's staff and clients for accuracy and noted where there are direct quotes from program staff or literature.

Chapter 3 defined four categories of health ministry and described the general ways the church has been involved in these areas.[2] The following descriptions are of several effective programs that illustrate three of these categories of health ministry. The liturgical/sacramental category will be illustrated in my future book, *Healing Liturgies for the Seasons of a Person's Life*. Hundreds of other models were researched that could not be included because of space constraints.

EDUCATIONAL

The Caring Network Volunteer Services

23 Magnolia Drive
New Providence, New Jersey 07974
Telephone: (908) 665-9829; fax: (908) 665-7941
Contact: Joanne Turner, Director

Mission and Activities. The Caring Network (CN) serves as an umbrella organization to support ministries "which engage in community restoration, healing and wholeness in order to live out the social message of the Bible." It links a number of faith communities together, be they Methodist or Jewish, "liberal" or "conservative," "Pentecostal" or "non-charismatic," in order to jointly support projects that build community in the wider sense of healing as *shalom*. The Network logo of a spiral emanating from a cross suggests a Christ-centered ministry that propels the church into the community and attracts the community to the church. It supports two main projects: (1) the Caring Community, Interfaith Caregivers (CCIC), a direct health care services project offering support to homebound persons in central New Jersey; and (2) the Central Jersey Parish Nursing Network (CJPN), a resource referral center for churches and institutions interested in starting parish nurse–based health ministries. The Prayer Net involves approximately fifty volunteers who pray daily, and some of them meet one hour per week for corporate prayer to uplift the Network's efforts.

Sponsors. Each of the two projects identified above has its own church and community sponsors. The Caring Community, Interfaith Caregivers operates out of a church office donated by the New Providence United Methodist Church. Ecumenical sponsors include six churches from a variety of denominations, a Jewish temple and community center, and county and health care organizations.

The CJPN is sponsored by a number of churches, community organizations, and individuals as well as the medical centers in Somerset and Muhlenberg.

Governance. Each project has its own board of directors comprised of sponsoring organizations. The CJPN has six volunteer positions: president, vice president, secretary, treasurer, membership coordinator, and program coordinator. Ad hoc committees are formed to plan local symposia on parish nursing.

Financial Support. The CCIC currently has an annual budget of about $5,000, which covers operating costs such as telephone, mailing, volunteer training, and volunteer insurance. Funds are received from local foundation grants, individual donations from both volunteers and "special friends," and money from churches and fund-raising events to cover the costs for the Caring Community.

The CJPN annual budget is less than $10,000. Funds for the CJPN are derived from membership dues from individuals, congregations, and institutions, and from program fees for spring and fall conferences.

Composition of Staff. The CCIC and the CJPN have one volunteer staff member, Joanne Turner, who oversees volunteer operations (fifty volunteers from local congregations who respond to the needs of about four clients per week) and also serves as director of the parent organization.

Persons Served. The CCIC serves homebound and infirm persons in Summit, New Providence, and Berkeley Heights, New Jersey. The CJPN serves churches and institutions that want to establish parish nurse–based ministries in central New Jersey. There are about forty participating congregations and three hundred parish nurses in the Network.

Types of Services. *Liturgical.* The CJPN offers models of healing and wholeness liturgies.

Educational. For the Caring Community, each of the sponsoring churches has a volunteer coordinator who has been trained by Joanne

Turner to offer nonprofessional services to the homebound. The coordinators in turn train volunteers from their church.

The CJPN is primarily a resource center that refers churches that want to begin a parish nursing program to other area churches that have already implemented such a program. "It defines the function of a parish nurse as a health educator, counselor, community resource agent, advocate and hands-on practitioner of health care in the church setting." Besides its role as a resource, it offers educational programs and support for nurses interested in parish nursing and compiles and disseminates health education materials for congregations.

It also provides information about parish nurse job descriptions, role expectations, insurance, and reporting structures to churches and organizations wishing to employ a parish nurse.

Support/Advocacy. The CCIC volunteers offer nonprofessional services to the homebound. These include providing reassurance by telephone, friendly visiting, shopping, running errands, and providing transportation to appointments.

Background and History. Joanne Turner founded the Caring Network. She left a full-time position as a clinical nurse specialist for critical care education at a university hospital in New York. When she read an ad about a $23 million Faith-in-Action grant in a professional nursing journal, the idea was born. She approached her pastor at the New Providence Presbyterian Church and talked to him about the possibility of seeking funds to start a health ministry. The two of them contacted other local ministers to brainstorm how they might combine their efforts so the entire community could benefit from such a grant.

This group of clergy met for more than a year, drawing on the expertise of community development leaders whom they invited as guest speakers at their meetings. By 1993, the group had solidified the bylaws and secured an initial grant of $25,000 from Faith-in-Action. The funds covered Turner's salary for eighteen months to spearhead the first effort of care for the homebound. However, her vision was greater; consequently, CN was incorporated in 1994 to allow expansion into parish nursing in 1995.

Overcoming Obstacles and Challenges. The ongoing challenge for Joanne Turner is finding enough volunteers to sustain the CCIC service for the homebound and being able to provide ongoing volunteer support. "If I can't give the volunteers attention, they just disappear," she says. It has been easier to keep volunteers for the CJPN because the volunteer nurses are already trained in their profession and therefore need little guidance once they have been given reference materials.

Another challenge for Turner is developing a working board of directors. "I have wonderful people but they need to be led," she explains. The full weight of the CN and its projects falls on her shoulders. She cannot be all things to all people as she balances a regular job with her family life and the demands of her volunteer directorship. "It's an ongoing challenge," she says, "to find sufficient time."

Chamblee-Doraville Ministry Center

5935 New Peachtree Road
Doraville, Georgia 30340
Telephone: (770) 451-1030; fax: (770) 451-6465
Contact: Rev. Samuel Bandela, Executive Director; Jean Murphy,
    Director of Health Ministries

Mission and Activities. The Chamblee-Doraville Ministry Center (CDMC) is a collaborative ministry effort among churches in the Atlanta area. The Interfaith Health Program (IHP), one of ten programs carried out by the ministry center, is a result of the collaboration of the Carter Center, Saint Joseph's Congregational Health Ministry program, and the Chamblee-Doraville Ministry Center itself. The IHP is composed of a coalition of twenty-five churches from different faiths and denominations; they are multiethnic, including Hispanic, Vietnamese, Chinese, and Korean congregations. The center operates a food pantry, a Bible club program, after-school tutoring programs, classes for English as a second language, a resource pregnancy center, and an annual health fair in areas of low-income housing.

Sponsors. Interdenominational support comes from more than twenty-five churches in the Atlanta area including Baptist, Lutheran, United Methodist, and Presbyterian.

Governance. CDMC is a 501(c)(3) organization that is managed by a nineteen-member board consisting of both men and women from five mainline denominations.

Financial Support. Funds come from churches and individuals.

Composition of Staff. There are eight staff positions: executive director; assistant director; programs director; directors of health ministries, church planting, and the Doraville Pregnancy Resource Center; food pantry aide; and chaplain. In addition, four hundred volunteers per year come primarily from Chamblee-Doraville churches.

Persons Served. Any person who is in need without discrimination based on religion, race, or faith in the greater Atlanta, Georgia, area. The ministry targets those living in zip codes 30340, 30360, 30341, and

30335, which are Doraville, Chamblee, and Buford corridor areas, to avoid duplication of services.

Types of Services. *Liturgical.* Through community outreach, the CDMC connects individuals as well as families to their choice of church in the community, or they are encouraged to attend church in one of the apartments under the CDMC church planting program.

Educational. Two parish nurses from Saint Joseph's Hospital are assigned to the CDMC; they work with thirty lay health promoters in twenty-five churches. The nurses and health promoters teach classes on living skills in the apartment complexes surrounding the center, conduct periodic health screenings, and work closely with other health agencies such as Mercy Mobile Health Care and Catholic Social Services. In addition, health education is facilitated in a variety of ways: church newsletters and bulletins, bulletin boards, brochures, health fairs, health forums on aging, CPR classes, stress management classes, health packets for children enrolled in local summer vacation Bible school programs, blood pressure and blood sugar screenings, parenting classes, and grief support groups.

Support/Advocacy. Provided by weekly and regular monthly meetings and seminars. People are referred to health clinics and hospitals for continued treatment and checkups where needed. Advocacy of public policy issues such as immigration laws, health care coverage, and other issues that impact the daily lives of this multiethnic population.

Background and History. The communities of Chamblee and Doraville in northern DeKalb County have experienced a cultural phenomenon in the past two decades. The Buford Highway Corridor has become metro Atlanta's undisputed magnet for immigrants, and the international population of this area has doubled in the past ten years. A group of committed Christians from four Baptist churches, seeing the challenges of adjustment for the newest neighbors, banded together to create a new ministry (CDMC) devoted initially to the unique needs of internationals.

With the arrival of Sam and Latha Bandela as the directors of the CDMC, the ministry expanded significantly. The Bandelas, now American citizens, are natives of India. They were appointed by Cooperative Baptist Fellowship as missionaries to serve the international community in Atlanta. From that humble beginning in February 1994, the CDMC has grown from four Baptist churches to thirty-five congregations of five mainline denominations; from two staff to eight full-time and one part-time; from two to seven days of program activities; from two to ten programs; and from a dozen to almost four hundred volunteers.

Overcoming Obstacles and Challenges. Developing cooperation and continuing support from pastors is an ongoing challenge. Fund-raising has been a continuing necessity after the initial grant. This is done by encouraging monthly donations; charging for training; and requesting donations from churches when doing a special project, for example, a health fair.

Presbyterian Health Education & Welfare Association (PHEWA)

100 Witherspoon Street
Louisville, Kentucky 40202-1396
Telephone: (502) 569-5794; fax: (502) 569-8034; E-mail:
  helenl@ctr.pcusa.org
Contact: Helen Locklear, Executive Director, PHEWA

Mission and Activities. PHEWA, a voluntary membership organization created by the General Assembly in 1956, is dedicated to the enactment of social justice and welfare ministries; it has ten networks that address particular concerns, some of which are organized around advocacy and support or persons with special health-related concerns. Its purpose is to provide resources for Presbyterians involved in social justice ministries. Its voluntary members are able to connect with other like-minded people in ministry, gain access to resources for ministry, and attend regional and national events for training. Modest membership fees of $35 ($25 PHEWA and $10 designated network) are charged to cover costs of the newsletter and other benefits. In 1998 the networks consisted of Presbyterian Health Network, Presbyterian AIDS Network, Presbyterian Network on Alcohol and Other Drug Use, Presbyterian Disabilities Concerns, Presbyterian Serious Mental Illness Network, Presbyterians Affirming Reproductive Options, Community Ministries and Neighborhood Organizations, Presbyterian Association of Specialized Pastoral Ministries, Presbyterian Child Advocacy Network, and Urban Presbyterian Pastors' Association. It raises the awareness level of the Presbyterian Church about the needs of marginalized groups, social justice issues, and health concerns affecting all peoples.

Presbyterian Health Network of PHEWA

Contact: Terrill L. Stumpf, Moderator

By way of illustration of one of PHEWA's networks, the rest of this description pertains to Presbyterian Health Network (PHN).

Mission and Activities. PHN "is a gathering of persons who affirm that the mission of the church fundamentally involves a call to ministries of health and healing, and who affirm the efforts of the Presbyterian Church (U.S.A.) to foster and promote health and healing ministries in its Congregations, Presbyteries, Synods, and General Assembly. The network encourages the Presbyterian Church (U.S.A.) at all its levels to develop and sustain a wide variety of health programs and ministries; foster critical ethical and theological reflection of health issues; and, unite Presbyterians in prayer and support for each other and the church in fulfilling their call to health and healing ministry."

Sponsor. Presbyterian Church (USA) in partnership with its Office of Health Ministries, staffed by Dave Zuverink and James Tippett.

Governance. An elected board from the Presbyterian Church constituents.

Financial Support. Presbyterian Church (USA) mission and selected budget. The 1997 budget was $37,050 for the Health Network. Expenses included team meetings, two national training events on parish nursing, and communication costs. A portion of the Presbyterian Health Network's income is derived from individual membership fees ($35).

Composition of Staff. An executive director, program assistant, meeting planner, child advocacy staff, outside consultants, and volunteer committee.

Persons Served. All Presbyterian churches and their surrounding communities in the United States.

Types of Services. *Liturgical.* PHN, in cooperation with the Office of Health Ministries, USA, has developed various worship resources, for example, a sample service of prayer and anointing with oil as well as a commissioning service of pastoral caregivers and health professionals to recognize and empower individuals in ministry.

Educational. PHN promotes education by developing curricula that model healthy structures and congregational policy for use in the local church and for health seminars and retreats for clergy and church professionals.

It provides materials that show churches how to develop a parish nurse program or a health ministry program that helps congregations make life-saving and life-enhancing choices in three areas: not smoking, sustaining good nutrition, and exercising. At the suggestion of PHN, the Board of Pensions offers the *Healthwise Handbook* for local churches to help "cut medical costs among its members and encourage better self care."

Support/Advocacy. PHN advocates for better public health policy at local, state, and federal government levels, works to interpret the needs of the marginalized, and raises ethical issues involving health and medicine.

Information is available to help churches become involved in political action and advocacy for a better national health care plan based on theological values from the Reformed tradition. These values underlie the ethical criteria for a national health care plan: caring; doing justice; preventing illness, curing and building community; stewardship; and community.

To help church professionals and their families cope with the stress of their ministry, lose weight, gain balance between their work and spiritual life, and other issues peculiar to ministry; PHN, the Office of Health Ministries, the Board of Pensions, the Synod of the Covenant, and others have prepared a *Staywell Program Handbook* designed to be used by synods, presbyteries, or groups of churches. It is user-friendly and easily adapted to different settings.

Direct Health Services. Preventive health tools such as the "Health Risk Appraisal" (HRA) help people learn about their major health risks and the choices that are available to improve health. It is a simple and inexpensive paper-and-pencil form that is easily filled out and returned with a personal interpretation of health status and major risks.

Overcoming Challenges and Obstacles. Interpreting and understanding the nature of this ministry to the church at large. It may be one of the best-kept secrets of the Presbyterian Church, and broadening its constituency and support is an ongoing effort.

Stephen Ministries

2045 Innerbelt Business Center Drive
St. Louis, Missouri 63114-5765
Telephone: (314) 428-2600; fax: (314) 428-7888
Web site: www.stephenministries.org
Contact: Dr. Kenneth Haugk, Executive Director; Rev. David Papp,
   Program Director

Mission and Activities. Stephen Ministries (SM) is a not-for-profit religious educational organization that provides resources for congregations to equip laypeople to provide quality ministry. Its mission is "to proclaim through word and deed the gospel of Jesus Christ by nurturing, edifying, educating, and equipping the whole people of God who are called, gifted and sent to be more effective servants who care for the needs of the whole person." Its primary resource is the Stephen Series, a system for organizing and equipping laypersons to provide one-to-one caring ministry to individuals facing a life challenge or crisis (for example, grief, joblessness, hospitalization, terminal illness). The pastors and lay leaders who will direct the ministry in a congregation are trained at an SM seven-day course; six of these courses are held at hotel and college campus sites across the country each year. The pastors and lay leaders return from these courses and then train lay caregivers, called Stephen Ministers, in their congregations. SM also offers the ChristCare Series system of small group ministry, as well as courses in evangelism, inactive member ministry, spiritual gifts, Christian caregiving, and dealing with church antagonism.

Sponsors. Transdenominational, international. "Over 7,000 congregations and organizations representing 80 denominations," primarily in the United States and Canada but also eighteen other countries on six continents.

Governance. Board of directors.

Financial Support. The annual budget of more than $1 million is covered by revenues from the one-time enrollment fee of $1,675 per church, conference fees, and other sources.

Composition of Staff. The total staff of fifty includes a ten-member pastoral and executive staff—including executive director, directors of project development, training courses, administration, human resources, and communications. Twenty-six volunteer staff assist the Stephen Ministries teaching faculty in seven-day training courses.

Persons Served. People in churches and surrounding communities primarily in the United States and Canada, but also in eighteen other countries on six continents, "who face the myriad challenges of life and may be bereaved, elderly, lonely, discouraged, terminally ill, home-bound, in a job or spiritual crisis, facing life transitions, separated or divorced, new church members or inactive members, single parents, experiencing the birth of a child—and many more stressful situations."

Types of Services. *Educational.* To train Stephen Leaders, congregations send one or more representatives to a seven-day Stephen Series Leader's Training Course, which is held in various locations, to learn how to implement and direct Stephen Ministry. Congregations pay a one-time enrollment fee of $1,675 (in 2000) for the training materials, regular updates, and ongoing support and consultation. Double occupancy conference fees, which include lodging and a number of meals, are under $800.

Once trained, the Stephen Leaders return to their churches to build awareness and ownership of Stephen Ministry in the congregation. They recruit and select laypeople for a minimum of fifty hours of training. The ongoing cycle of recruiting, training, referring, and supervising laypeople keeps the program in motion to meet the caring ministry needs as defined by each church and community.

"The training is designed to be easy to understand, but in-depth. Training materials are two-tiered." One set is designed for the Stephen Leaders and includes "2,200 pages of teaching and administrative materials in a file folder system for easy reference," experiential exercises, and extensive skill practicing instructions. The second set (400 pages long) is for the lay caregivers being trained by the Stephen Leaders, based on life situations and sample dialogues for discussion and skill practice.

Background and History. Stephen Ministries was founded in 1975 by Dr. Kenneth C. Haugk, a pastor and clinical psychologist who saw more needs for care in his congregation and community than he alone as pastor could provide. He began training laypersons to assist in providing distinctively Christian care. The ministry was so successful in his congregation that other churches became interested, and Haugk founded the Stephen Ministries organization.

As Reverend Haugk tells the story, the eight people he selected were a "typical church conglomeration made up of a secretary, a teacher, a homemaker, a student, a director of public relations, a small business owner, an insurance agent, and a retired beautician. All had responded positively to my invitation: 'We're going to start a caring ministry here where people care for others one-to-one. I'm going to begin some training in January. Would you like to be part of that?' I didn't do any arm-twisting. Eight out of the ten people I asked said yes. They probably weren't all that surprised to be asked. I had made no secret of my interest in training lay people for caring since my arrival in this St. Louis church. The class went well enough. We had our commissioning service in March (Amazing! Lay people were willing to give three months just for training!). I had people all lined up who were in need of ministry: A man whose wife had recently died. Someone who was blind—she wasn't even a member of the congregation. Lighthouse for the Blind had heard what we were doing and wondered if we had someone who could visit her. A young woman with cancer. A shut-in. An inactive member who was struggling with his faith. A truck driver who had to retire early because of two heart attacks.

"Around the time of the second supervisory session, in our follow-up time together, something clicked with those first Stephen Ministers. They listened to each other's practical concerns. They witnessed the ministry that was happening. An awareness took off like a fire among them: 'We really are helping! We're ministering! We're meeting the needs of hurting people.' I refrained from saying, 'Of course.'

"That spring at a party for the caregivers and their families, the small business owner and the teacher cornered me. 'This is too good to keep to ourselves,' she said. 'You've got to share this with other congregations,' he said. 'Yes, you're right,' I said. But I didn't do anything about it. I was happy just supervising this first caring team.

"A month or so later our paths crossed again, this time at church. It was a hot May day, sweltering in fact. No air-conditioning, and I was still robed in my vestments. The teacher and the small business owner backed me against a wall and left me with no escape! They literally sweated a promise out of me! I had to make the training available to some other local congregations. And the rest, as they say, is history."

Overcoming Obstacles and Challenges. The biggest challenge for the Stephen Series has been overcoming many congregations' belief that the caring ministry is exclusively "the pastor's job." The pastor continues to provide caring ministry in a Stephen Series congregation, but also becomes an "equipper," helping to inspire, train, and lead laypersons to provide substantive Christian care. The expanded caregiving ministry through Stephen Ministry shows how cost-effective Stephen Ministry can be when compared to the cost of hiring additional church staff persons to increase the caregiving capacity of a congregation.

The Stephen Series also challenges the paradigm that laypeople will not make a major time commitment to ministry. (Stephen Ministers make a two-year commitment involving fifty hours of initial training, weekly visits with a care receiver, and twice monthly supervision and continuing education sessions.) More than 250,000 laypersons have been trained and have served as Stephen Ministers since 1975. Tens of thousands of others have committed a week or more to attend a Leader's Training Course in order to be trained as Stephen Leaders so that they can work with their pastors to direct the congregation's Stephen Ministry.

World Council of Churches (WCC)

Mission and Evangelism Team Health and Healing Work (successor
   to Christian Medical Commission)
150 Route de Ferney
1211 Geneva 2, Switzerland
Telephone: 0041-22-791 61 11; fax: 0041-22-791 03 61; Web site:
   <http://www.wcc-coe.org>
Contact: Dr. Manoj Kurian

Mission and Activities of WCC. Consultations and activities in mission and evangelism, health and healing, are offered to equip and strengthen churches in mission. The concern of WCC is to make clear God's loving, eternal purpose to heal and reconcile all people to God in Jesus Christ and to restore wholeness to all creation. The health ministries are now carried out by the Mission and Evangelism Team.

Sponsors of WCC. More than 330 churches in 100 countries.

Governance of WCC. The Assembly of the WCC member churches, which meets approximately every seven years, is the supreme legislative body. Between assemblies, the Central Committee guides the work of the Secretariate.

Financial Support of the Mission and Evangelism Team. The work of the Mission and Evangelism Team is supported through membership dues and donations from member churches to WCC and funds received from individuals, church organizations, and agencies for development—many of whom are government based but work in accordance with Christian aims.

Composition of Staff of the Mission and Evangelism Team. A nine-member team, two of whom have special responsibility for the health and healing aspects of the WCC mission.

Persons Served by the Health and Healing Work. Those recognized, particularly by member churches, as being appropriate recipients of the service toward health and healing enabled by the team.

Types of Services. *Educational.* The work of the team promotes adult education for personal empowerment and social transformation. It also promotes reflective and practical education for various aspects of community involvement in health. This work is furthered by the publication of *Contact*, an international magazine, produced in India and Latin America four times a year. It reports topical, innovative, and courageous approaches to the promotion of health and integrated development. It is available in English, French, Spanish, Portuguese, and Chinese.

Support/Advocacy. The team advocates policies that encourage equitable sharing and rational investment in drugs and medical equipment, strengthens networks of health care coordinating agencies, and promotes and monitors the development of sustainable church health institutions and programs. It represents the Christian voice and values, as well as facilitates and advocates for justice in health policy making and service distribution. In this way, it makes connections with major international agencies, such as WHO, UNICEF, and NGO Forum for Health.

Direct Health Services. Help is offered to member churches in their ministries of health, healing, and wholeness. Community-based health care and training and the work of equipping churches to meet the challenge of HIV/AIDS are two important examples.

Background and History. The WCC was founded by representatives of 147 churches in 1948. The more than 330 WCC member churches today include Orthodox churches, historic Protestant denominations such as Anglican, Baptist, Lutheran, Methodist, and Reformed, and a broad representation of independent churches. The Roman Catholic Church (RCC) is not a member of the WCC, but maintains close collaboration and fraternal solidarity with the council in several areas, including being a full member of the WCC's Faith and Order Commission and RCC/WCC Joint Working Group, a well-established consultative forum.

In 1964 and 1968 ecumenical consultations organized in Tubingen, Germany, jointly by the WCC and the Lutheran World Federation focused on medical missions in the Third World and the church's role in healing. The Christian Medical Commission (CMC) was created within the WCC in 1968 to assist the member churches to deal with questions being raised about these subjects and to encourage church-related health programs to develop ecumenical cooperation.

During CMC's early years, emphasis was placed on promotion of primary health care as a means of redressing the imbalance between this and more sophisticated, expensive institutional medical care. Primary health care became a global movement adopted by all World Health Organization members at a conference that CMC helped to organize in 1978.

During the same period, however, growing dissatisfaction with the so-called garage-mechanic approach in modern medicine made Christian groups in many countries begin to search for health care that more fully addressed the needs of the whole person. The CMC embarked on a program to study health, healing, and wholeness at the grassroots. Regional consultations in Trinidad, Honduras, Botswana, India, Indonesia, Papua New Guinea, Ecuador, United States, Hungary, and Japan brought together more than eight hundred pastors, theologians, and health workers to discuss the Christian perspective of health. (As part of the U.S. gathering, I found this consultation inspirational.)

In July 1989, in Moscow, the final report was presented to the Central Committee. The study affirmed clearly that health is not primarily medical and identified the spiritual dimension as particularly important.

CMC was renamed CMC-Churches' Action for Health in a primary reorganization of the WCC, and then the health ministry was moved in 1999 under the Mission and Evangelism Team of WCC. The work of assisting churches around the world to address health issues as a demonstration of God's love and concern for the whole person is now undertaken by the Mission Team. They are assisted by a network of ecumenical Christian health associations.

SUPPORT/ADVOCACY

Food & Friends

58 L Street SE
Washington, D.C. 20003

Telephone: (202) 488-8278; fax: (202) 488-1521
Contact: Craig Shniderman, Executive Director; Mickie Ballotta,
   Development Director

Mission and Activities. The goal of Food & Friends (F&F) is delivery of
hot, nutritious food at no cost to people living with AIDS in the greater
Washington, D.C., area who are fighting to maintain their health and independence. Each Monday through Saturday, hundreds of volunteers deliver 3
meals at midday to sustain clients with a healthy diet. About 15,000 meals
(7 different diets) are served to 950 clients weekly. These meals include food
that is previously prepared and frozen, and groceries. In addition, nutrition
assessment and counseling, cooking classes, and dietary education workshops enable persons with AIDS to prepare their own meals.

Approximately 60 percent of the AIDS deaths that occur annually in
the United States are linked to dietary problems. A regular nutritious diet
is a strong weapon against AIDS. That is why F&F is dedicated solely to
delivering quality meals to the HIV/AIDS population and is not trying to
meet all the needs of persons with AIDS, of which there are 45,000 in metropolitan D.C.

Sponsors. Originally founded by a Presbyterian minister, F&F is no
longer formally affiliated with the church. It is aligned with a wide variety
of community groups, businesses, and religious organizations, and it is
supported by individuals, foundations, and congregations.

Governance. A self-perpetuating board of directors consisting of physicians, attorneys, business owners and managers, clergy, and government
leaders.

Financial Support. An annual budget of $4 million from foundations
and individuals (75 percent) and from Ryan White government grants
(25 percent). Twenty-five percent is applied to administrative and fund-
raising expenses.

Composition of Staff. Fifty staff (seven part-time and forty-three
full-time), which include a full-time director, administrative and development staff, nutritionists, cooks, drivers, and other support staff. In
addition, five hundred volunteers per week annually contribute $432,000
worth of services.

Persons Served. Daily deliveries are made to persons with AIDS and
their families living in a 750-square-mile area, including the District of
Columbia, suburban Maryland, and northern Virginia; clients in another
4,550-square-mile area receive deliveries of groceries and frozen entrees.
Clients are referred by health care facilities or come through self-referral.
The profile of the recipients is 80 percent African American, 5 percent

Latino, 15 percent Caucasian; 40 percent female, 60 percent male, including 175 children. F&F estimates that it adds 60 new clients each month. The client number grew to 950 in 1998; this will result in an additional 150,000 meals in 1999.

Types of Services. *Educational.* The Nutrition Education & Support Project provides clients with nutritional assessments and counseling by a licensed staff dietitian; nutrition and AIDS education materials and workshops; and cooking classes for people with AIDS and their caregivers.

Support/Advocacy. Indirectly through participation in organizations such as AIDS Action Council and AIDS Nutrition Services Alliance.

Direct Health Services. Serving hot meals daily.

Background and History. F&F was started in 1988 in the basement of Westminster Presbyterian Church in Washington, D.C., to deliver free, freshly prepared meals to homebound people with AIDS. With the vision of Rev. Carla Gorrell, Presbyterian minister at Westminster Presbyterian Church, and some financial support and space from the church, as well as church member volunteers, F&F has grown from the original handful of volunteers serving 30 clients a day to 500 volunteers serving about 1,000 clients weekly. Under the leadership of Craig Shniderman, who became director four years ago, they moved into a 19,000-square-foot building including a 3,000-square-foot kitchen.

Shniderman, a health care administrator with extensive fund-raising and administrative experience with nonprofits, is the right person to carry the vision forward. In the future, as the AIDS epidemic decreases, the organization may look to serve other ill clients with nutritional needs.

Overcoming Obstacles and Challenges. The greatest initial difficulty for this ministry was fear and ignorance about AIDS. Since it was started by a small Presbyterian church, the major resource was volunteers, not money. Through the perseverance of its founder, funding, a facility, and more volunteers were secured. Under its current director a decaying warehouse was transformed into a beautiful building with colorful walls and pictures. This multicolored facility sits in the midst of decaying warehouses in one of the poorer neighborhoods of D.C.-Anacostia. It is true that there is no need for an organization to look poor just because it serves the poor. As Shniderman states, "Keeping focused on our central mission, even in light of other pressing and important needs, is the reason for our success." One of the biggest challenges facing most social services and nonprofits is becoming too diffuse. Success, believes the staff, is measured by *how* they deliver the meals, which is as important as the meals themselves. Being reliable and accessible, offering friendship and family-centered care, and seeking wellness and independence for their clients are the priorities.

Point Loma/Ocean Beach Respite Care Network

Point Loma Community Presbyterian Church
2128 Chatsworth Boulevard
San Diego, California 92107
Telephone: (619) 223-7753; fax: (619) 223-7753 (call before
    sending fax)
Contact: JoAnn Bitner, Director; Kathleen Grove, Chairman of
    the Board

Mission and Activities. The Point Loma/Ocean Beach Respite Care
Network (PLRCN) is an ecumenical service program that matches volunteers with caregivers to provide them a regular break from their duties in
attending a homebound loved one with a chronic health care problem such
as Alzheimer's disease. The Network provides four hours per week of free
in-home companionship for elderly adults for a minimum of one year so
that their primary caretakers can get out of the house to relax or attend to
personal matters. Some caregivers are supporting an infirm spouse; others
are tending to elderly parents. One goal of the program is to keep the loved
one at home as long as possible.

In addition to the PLRCN, this very active church of 2,100 members
is involved in other health ministries. A physician comes to the church
once a week to offer basic health education to congregation members, and
a Stephen Ministry has been implemented.

Sponsors. Point Loma Community Presbyterian Church and Xerox
Corporation.

Governance. The five-member board of directors is composed of two
sociologists, an attorney, a business executive from Xerox Corporation, an
M.D. geriatrics specialist, and the director ex officio.

Financial Support. The Network began with a $17,000 grant and now
has an annual budget of approximately $10,000 contributed by the Xerox
Corporation and Presbyterian Women Thank Offering. An entrepreneur-
ial payment system has been set up; the director is remunerated for her
services in relation to the number of volunteers she recruits and trains and
the number of recipients she locates: $50 for every volunteer; $50 for every
recipient; and $1 an hour for each hour of contact between the volunteers
and the families to whom they provide companioinship.

Composition of Staff. There is one part-time director, JoAnn Bitner, who has
a Ph.D. in family counseling. She has trained thirty-three active volunteers.

Persons Served. Elderly and homebound adults with chronic health care
problems not needing nursing-level services in Point Loma and Ocean

Beach communities of San Diego. Respite care is offered in the homes of the people receiving care. Volunteers' training and administration are based at Point Loma Community Presbyterian Church. The program has served more than forty-two families to date.

Types of Services. *Educational.* Volunteers receive an initial half-day training by the program director, and then monthly in-service training for two hours in the evening when they talk about their experience and raise questions. In addition, mini courses in stress reduction and other topics are offered.

Support/Advocacy. As respite is provided to the caregiver, the Network also strives to offer companionship for the person who is receiving care. Counseling on an informal basis through "active listening" is at times offered by volunteers; the director always meets with the family first to see if respite care is appropriate.

Visits to the homes of families receiving respite care reveal the bond of friendship that develops between the volunteer and the family. It is a bond engendered over the four hours per week (typically 9:00 A.M. to 1:00 P.M.) during the year to which the volunteer commits. The volunteers are not to cook or clean or necessarily give medications. They may assist the patient to walk around the house, but really they are viewed as companions. Clearly, they find the role fulfilling. One volunteer expresses her motivation: "I can do something where I am needed." Trust is a very important dimension and seems to emanate first from the connection with the church, the director, and then the volunteer.

Background and History. The visionary of the Respite Care Network was Kathleen Grove, a sociologist who teaches at the University of San Diego and is a member of Point Loma Presbyterian Church. Concerned by local statistics that showed a two-year waiting list for people to receive respite care services, Grove, who now chairs the board, began to discuss the need for respite care in 1993 with the church pastor and other members including Stephen Ministry volunteers. They decided upon a narrow focus of training volunteers to be companions for homebound elderly persons. The Network was launched in December 1995 after a mission statement was written, a prayer chain for the effort was established, and funding was secured.

Overcoming Obstacles and Challenges. The challenge facing caregivers is that most of them are also carrying full-time jobs, which is why Xerox Corporation stepped in to help fund the church-based effort. As members of the baby boomer generation face the hardships of caring for their aging parents, their employers are seeing the effects on their workforce. "Without help, caregivers can become physically and emotionally exhausted." What appealed to the church on a theological level also made sense to a corporation on the practical level of employee health. Curiously, there is a reticence on the part of family members to admit that they need assistance and caring for a spouse or a parent. They are reluctant to access the services of the Network for which one would expect a waiting list. This attitude may change as the program gains acceptance in the community over time.

For those who are participants in the program, there have been no complaints or legal issues raised, which is quite amazing considering the delicate care offered. The volunteers' sense of commitment has been one of the major reasons for the program's success. They are committed because of the payoff for them in being needed and belonging to their community; and because of the volunteer team-building and continuing education nurtured at the monthly meetings led by the program director.

In starting a respite care program like Point Loma's, one is advised to have a businessperson, a lawyer, and an M.D. on the board. This group assures that all issues have been addressed, such as waiver forms signed by the recipients of care. A full written description of the program was sent to the church's insurance company, which indicated that the church's existing policy would cover the ministry without additional coverage.

(RAIN) Regional AIDS Interfaith Network—Arkansas

P.O. Box 3776
Little Rock, Arkansas 72203
Telephone: (800) 851-6301; fax: (501) 376-6036
Contact: Sybil Cunningham, Interim Director

Mission and Activities. RAIN is a national interfaith movement founded and sponsored by the Interfaith Alliance of Arkansas—an ecumenical, interfaith network of communities of faith in Arkansas. All interfaith AIDS agencies are independent from one another. RAIN affirms that "God wills dignity and fullness of life for ALL persons; that illness, suffering and death are part of the mystery of living; that God is especially present to those who are alienated, oppressed or misunderstood; that AIDS is NOT God's punishment for sin, and that God stands by, and will continue to stand by, people with AIDS." The following by way of example is a description of the Arkansas chapter.

RAIN—Arkansas is a statewide network of 126 congregation-based Care Teams (CTs) with more than 1,700 trained volunteers in 14 denominations, which RAIN has recruited and trained. CTs provide direct support services and pastoral care for persons with HIV/AIDS, their families, and caregivers.

Care Teams have a minimum of seven members, consisting of men and women ranging in age from fourteen to eighty-five who are students, professionals, retirees, homemakers, and individuals from diverse social and economic backgrounds. After extensive training, CTs are connected with Care Partners (persons with HIV/AIDS) and their families. Care Partners reflect the great diversity of persons infected with the HIV virus: heterosexual and homosexual individuals and couples, infants and single mothers, families, homeless persons, children, and recovering addicts. CTs help persons with HIV/AIDS to "live longer with AIDS" and "to die with dignity." They achieve this by home and hospital visitations, food preparation and service, nonskilled nursing care, grief counseling, prayer, nonjudgmental emotional and spiritual support, shopping, transportation to doctors' offices and errands, and referrals to health care and other resources. As Care Partners live longer and are more physically able to care for themselves most of the time, Care Teams and Care Partners alike share their love, friendship, and fellowship, and experience "family bonding."

Sponsors. An interfaith mix of congregations from fourteen denominations.

Governance. The board of directors of RAIN includes persons with HIV/AIDS, doctors, lawyers, clergy, and other lay professionals and volunteers.

Financial Support. RAIN receives financial support from foundations (especially Levi-Strauss, Robert Wood Johnson Local Funding Partner Initiative), churches, synagogues, individuals, and specific fund-raising activities. RAIN's 1998 annual budget was $499,000, of which 27 percent came from gifts, 1 percent from fees, 1 percent from United Way, 1 percent from product sales, 32 percent from fund-raising events, 18 percent from grants, and 20 percent from churches and miscellaneous sources.

Composition of Staff. An executive director, eight other full-time employees, and eleven regional consultants who receive a small monthly stipend. Annually, there are 1,700 RAIN volunteers serving in Care Teams of seven to twenty-five members.

Persons Served. From newborn infants with AIDS to senior citizens with AIDS in Arkansas.

Types of Services. *Liturgical.* Sponsoring of worship services, including World AIDS Day (December 1) Memorial Services. When a Care Partner dies, the corresponding Care Team attends a Rainbow Retreat, which is an opportunity in the words of the participants to "heal their grief and anger and sadness" and "help them say good-bye" so they can meet and care for a new Care Partner. Four-day Heartsong Spiritual Retreats for more than forty-five men and women living with HIV/AIDS are held twice a year.

Educational. Recognizing that education and prevention are the only vaccines for HIV/AIDS, RAIN sponsors education programs throughout Arkansas for high schools, middle schools, churches and faith groups, healthcare providers, civic groups, community groups, and even in local Wal-Mart stores. These presentations and courses feature current statistics about HIV/AIDS, personal stories of people affected by HIV/AIDS, and lectures on codependency, pastoral care, updates on new medications, treatments, and drug abuse. RAIN also offers continuing education, grief counseling, and spiritual support to Care Teams. RAIN also hosts two wellness weekends per year in collaboration with the Ryan White Center. Care Teams are maintained through monthly team meetings, monthly meetings for team leaders, and quarterly in-service education and memorial days.

Support/Advocacy. In cooperation with the Ryan White Center and other local and national AIDS organizations, RAIN participates in advocacy programs in Little Rock and Washington, D.C., and works closely with social work services.

Background and History. In 1989, Margaret Austin, an Episcopal chaplain in New Orleans, in cooperation with Associated Catholic Charities in New Orleans, received a grant from the Robert Wood Johnson Foundation to pilot a two-year, four-state project on interfaith AIDS education and prevention. The four states were Arkansas, Texas, Louisiana, and Oklahoma. Soon after, the Religious Advisory Committee of the AIDS Foundation began to develop the groundwork for RAIN. This advisory committee included well-known laypeople and clergy, such as Rev. Norwood Jones, an HIV-positive Methodist minister and community leader. Also in 1989, RAIN hired its first employee and trained its first Care Team at Christ Episcopal Church in Little Rock, followed by Care Teams at St. James Methodist, Second Presbyterian, Temple B'nai Israel, and St. Mark's Episcopal congregations in Little Rock. In 1991, with seventeen Care Teams in active ministry and at the end of its first grant, RAIN increased its financial base. It changed its governance from that of an advisory committee to a board of directors, and hired its second employee. In 1992, RAIN secured nonprofit status, became independent of the AIDS Foundation, and began regional expansion.

Overcoming Obstacles and Challenges. Pat Camp, an Arkansas RAIN volunteer, identified three obstacles with which RAIN continues to struggle. All three obstacles relate directly to the cultural myths and misunderstandings surrounding HIV/AIDS. Namely, local municipalities and faith congregations often deny that there are persons with HIV/AIDS who need care in their area. Most churches identify "caring for people living with AIDS" as "promoting the homosexual lifestyle." Finally, fear is the predominant emotion of both individuals infected and individuals affected by HIV/AIDS. Those infected with HIV or who are living with AIDS often fear rejection by friends, family members, and their communities if they share their need for help. Many uninfected individuals live in fear of contagion from ministry with persons with AIDS, even when there exists no possibility of transmission (e.g., through a handshake, hospital visit, and so forth). Camp saw prayer combined with RAIN's educational programs as two important means to overcoming these obstacles. Through prayer, RAIN staff members and volunteers "waited on God" and prayed that God would draw enough people together to form Care Teams in various areas.

Like so many others, Camp overcame denial, processed her fear, and separated homosexuality from the pandemic of AIDS through personal interaction with people living with AIDS. "We became active when our youngest son was diagnosed HIV-positive in January 1992 and developed AIDS in November 1992," shares Camp. "We witnessed first hand what families and PWAs here go through—the journey is hard to walk alone." Camp concludes, "RAIN's goal is to prevent any other families from walking alone and to walk alongside others who have been touched by this monster called AIDS that has already claimed too many of our young people."

DIRECT HEALTH SERVICES

Bethel Baptist Healing Ministry

Bethel Baptist Church
6 Hope Road
Kingston 10, Jamaica
Contact: Mr. Raemil Lewis, Director; Dr. Anthony Allen,
     Consultant—Mission and Activities

Mission and Activities. The Bethel Baptist Healing Ministry (BBHM) is a model of health delivery that seeks to reverse the influence of mind/body dualism and materialism, which have limited the effectiveness of Western scientific medicine; it examines the underlying problems of illness rather than offering simply a shot or a pill. In addition, the Bethel community has learned through sharing sessions and personal struggles that even those in the ministry of healing are in need of healing. They are dependent on the empowerment and daily guidance of God, who loves us, makes us whole, and binds us together.[3] The ministry now offers more than twenty services including promotive, preventive, curative, and rehabilitative programs and community outreach. The management committee and staff of Bethel's Health Centre started a community outreach effort because they recognized that much of the illness they were seeing resulted from the social disorganization of the surrounding community. Services now include maternity monitoring, "well-child" clinics, family planning advice, health education, immunization, medical screening, and care for the elderly.

Sponsors. Bethel Baptist Church.

Governance. Church Council of Bethel Baptist Church.

Financial Support. Health Centre patients and counseling clients pay a fee based on their income. Since patients and clients are generally poor, their contributions cover about 25 percent of the ministry's expenses. In-kind contributions from Bethel Baptist Church cover another 50 percent of the costs. The remaining shortfall is covered by international funding agencies.

Composition of Staff. Nine full-time and nine part-time staff and more than one hundred church and community volunteers.

Persons Served. There are 2,000 Bethel Baptist Church members, 800 residents nearby in a low-income Kingston neighborhood, and approximately 5,000 people in three rural communities (for periodic promotive and preventive services).

Types of Services. *Liturgical.* A group meets weekly to pray for the sick, and Healing Sundays are held twice a year to emphasize divine healing as part of worship.

Educational. Preventive health education is offered in family planning, family life, care for the elderly, first aid, and ministering to persons with HIV/AIDS. In addition, lay leaders offer classes on preparation for retirement, aging, marriage, parenting, separation, divorce, and violence in the home. A healing ministry bibliography and other educational resources have been developed.

Support/Advocacy. Church members are divided into birth month "caring groups," who support each other in times of distress, celebrate in times of joy, and carry out small outreach projects. Each of these groups has a lay leader and team leader. Several laypersons receive training in counseling and basic health care promotion.

In addition, the management committee and staff of the Healing Centre have started a wholistic community outreach and "self organization" effort, recognizing that much of the illness they were seeing resulted from the social disorganization of the surrounding community.

Direct Health Services. The ministry's wholistic care center, called the Healing Centre, has grown into a three-story building attached to the church. New patients are screened by a nurse who notes mental, spiritual, social, and physiological concerns with the aid of a Wholistic Assessment Questionnaire. The patients are then referred to the Healing Centre's medical doctors, counseling psychologists, prayer counselors, and the church's social worker, as appropriate. Services include maternity monitoring, immunization, and medical screening. There is a church community nurse outreach service for the elderly, the mentally ill, and persons with HIV/AIDS.

Background and History. In 1972 Bethel Baptist Church Council explored the role of the church in healing by developing a ministry to the body, mind, and spirit of its members and the surrounding community. They were concerned with the lack of health care for the poor in Jamaica. Through the vision of pastor Burchell Taylor and physician Anthony Allen, the center grew and received outside funding from the Christian Medical Commission of the World Council of Churches, Bread for the World, and other organizations.

Overcoming Obstacles and Challenges. The Bethel Baptist community's first concern is about prolonged dependency on outside financial resources. The church council is exploring alternative sources of support such as increased tithing by church members, special donations by members and Friends of the Ministry, and income-generating activities. These have included the operation of a multipurpose pharmacy and sales outlet.

The community team also struggles to find patience and diligence in the face of slow uphill progress. Despite all its gains in the Ambrook Lane neighborhood, the majority of the people still lack jobs, adequate housing, and proper education. Drug addiction, violence, and mainly apathy from demoralization remain intractable problems. Party politics still divide. Brought together by migration and united chiefly by poverty, the squatters (in the area) have a formidable challenge to become a community of respected, liberated citizens. Nevertheless, a growing nucleus of community members have built an expanding basic school, formed a citizens association, and strengthened cooperation in areas such as sports, sanitation, skill training, and spiritual nurture.

The Bethel Model has been visited and observed by several churches over the years. After twenty-four years of operation, this healing community is encouraged that the "Healing Ministry Movement" has spread to all denominations in Jamaica.

Bromley by Bow Centre

1 Bruce Road, Bromley by Bow
London E3 3HN, England
Telephone: 0181-980-4618; fax: 0181-880-6608
Contact: Rev. Andrew Mawson, Chairman; Allison Trimble, Chief
    Executive, Bromley by Bow Centre

Mission and Activities. Bromley by Bow Centre (B by B or the Centre) is "a pioneering voluntary organization in the East End of London which seeks to improve the quality of life of local people." Arising out of "one of the most deprived areas in England, with multiple social problems," the Centre has discerned, nurtured, and helped to focus the "great reserves of energy and ability in the local community" and created a climate of encouragement and expectation. The projects evolve around five integrated "pillars" of the Centre: health and care, the arts, education and training, the environment, and enterprise. Through a "vibrant mix of activities" numbering more than 125 each week that involve more than two thousand people each week, the Centre aims at creating "effective social change . . . leading to a community of individuals able to engage with local issues and bring about their own transformations" and at lifting "low self-esteem by creating opportunities for excellence and achievement and to open up possibilities by encouraging people to dream."

Sponsors. The Centre began as a project of an old United Reformed Church. Although the Centre has grown to be independent, the church is "a core sanctuary around which the bustle of the Centre's activities revolve." The Centre has secured broad partnership and support from a range of corporations, charitable trusts and other charities, and the public sector. Its patrons are Lord Peyton of Yeovil and Lord Young of Dartington.

Governance. A management committee of twenty persons oversees B by B with the executive staff.

Financial Support. Government grants, charitable lottery funds, foundations, corporations, and the private sector. In December 1996, the Centre received $4.4 million over seven years from the British government's Single Regeneration Budget. The total core budget for 1997 was $1.2 million. The mortgage on the new Health Centre is "serviced by rent paid" by the general practitioners under the National Health Service who occupy part of the building.

Composition of Staff. There are sixty staff and tutors, and fifty volunteers. Centre activities are grouped into projects, each one run by a project manager.

Persons Served. In 1997, the Centre served 2000 persons per week of the following ethnicities: white (44 percent), Indian subcontinent (33 percent, primarily Bengali), black (14 percent), Chinese/Vietnamese (4 percent), other (5 percent). Two-thirds of those served are female.

Types of Services. *Educational.* More than 150 local people at any one time receive skill training to improve employment opportunities. The Centre's Taking Hold project, established through a three-year grant, helps young people from the community to start their own businesses by providing business training and overall support.

The Centre is a participant in a Lifelong Skills program (sponsored by Royal & Sun Alliance) that encourages good citizenship and helps quantify skills, such as communication, problem solving, team leadership, and social interaction. This program has assisted young people by providing needed skills and increasing their self-esteem.

The Sparks project, based around the Centre's Youth Project, is a collaboration of B by B, the Atomic Weapons Establishment at Aldermaston, the Institute of Child Health, and the Committee for the Public Understanding of Science. This project trains fourteen- to sixteen-year-olds in park design and improvement. The designs of these students for play equipment "themed around the body" have been successfully constructed. In 1997, the students were working on a collection of toys that supplement the equipment and help "teach about the body and health."

Bromley by Bow's Healthy Living Centre (HLC) provides "consultancy advice about community regeneration and HLCs to health professionals and voluntary groups" around England and Northern Ireland. It offers a series of seminars about HLCs for health authorities, voluntary groups, and others.

A day-long nursery, separately constituted but working in partnership with Bromley by Bow Church, provides care and activities for twenty-five children and their parents. Additional activities include stone carving, stop smoking seminars, Muslim Women's Bereavement Service, Bengali classes, multicultural groups, and other training programs.

Support/Advocacy. Advocacy for effective social change and excellence in Bromley by Bow and transformation and empowerment of individuals are motivating factors for all of the Centre's programs. Its philosophy is "one of mutuality, creativity and making connections between people and cultures."

With a holistic vision, the Centre's advocacy includes not only individuals but also the environment in which they live; it believes that the environment affects people's aspirations. The Centre enables horticultural professionals to restore "the neighborhood park, previously semi-derelict, as a beautiful public space." B by B's "Enterprise Zone," a bright space converted from a woodwork shop that had been Sunday school rooms in the 1970s, is being used by new enterprises and community businesses. It also sponsors housing projects.

Direct Health Services. In 1997 B by B completed a new Health Centre, the "first example of a community organization designing, building and owning a health center" in the United Kingdom; teams of nurses and doctors work not only with other health professionals but with artists and community workers. The Health Centre operates as a "Health Market Place" for patients to make their own health choices. These options include medical care, complementary therapies, and a broad range of "integrated activities which have a direct health gain, e.g. dance classes for large and luscious ladies (their choice of name), portrait painting for people with mental illness, silk painting for pregnant women who are drug dependent, and training local volunteers as health outreach workers."

The Health Centre also offers "community care" on weekdays to groups of elderly people and people with disabilities, with arts and health-related activities led by volunteers and trained professionals.

Background and History. B by B began in 1984 as a mission project of the twelve-member worshiping congregation of an old United Reformed Church. The church sanctuary and education buildings were transformed into a centre for community. In the center a tent/tabernacle is suspended from the ceiling over the altar and pews. The sanctuary's perimeter has been temporarily partitioned into sections for a nursery/day care center with activity areas, play equipment, and so forth. When a larger space is needed periodically for gatherings, the partitions are removed. The education building has been converted into a coffee house/restaurant, Pie in the Sky, which is self-supporting. There are pottery, sculpture, and craft studios where the products made are sold to generate funds for the Centre.

This project is the vision of the Bromley by Bow Church's pastor, Rev. Andrew Mawson. He was challenged by an empty church and a decaying inner-city community and saw his role as a social entrepreneur and the church as a catalyst for an emerging renaissance of the local community.

Mawson comments, "Our distinctive model of community development has grown from a theology which has sought to interpret the role of the church in the light of the complexity of the inner city and has tried to embrace that complexity without sentimentality or ideological compartmentalizing. The liturgical space has been redesigned and remains a core sanctuary around which the bustle of the day revolves. Like the medieval cathedral, the church sits amidst the market place of everyday activity, allowing the vibrancy and diversity of life to surround it and enabling a mutual crossover of influence between the secular and sacred."

Overcoming Obstacles and Challenges. Bromley by Bow is the second-most-deprived ward in the United Kingdom, with poor housing conditions and the highest density of population. It suffers from racism, poverty, and violence, as well as from generations of unemployment and lack of resources.

As might be expected, the health of the Bromley by Bow population is poor. Mortality rates from malignant cancers, TB, suicide, and poisoning are above the national average; psychiatric morbidity is high; drug abuse abounds; and 16.5 percent of the population suffers from a chronic illness. Traditional health care "does not acknowledge the range of people's physical, psychological and social needs." The Bromley by Bow Health Centre, however, understands "the interplay between health in the medical context and well-being in its broader setting." Its staff and volunteers recognize the need for "an integrated and holistic approach, and are working to evolve a model of healthcare that integrates solutions to what are essentially integrated problems." The Centre as a whole believes that an organic model is critical to its development, "starting small, not necessarily following a grand plan but allowing things to take shape as a pragmatic response to need." Yet "results have been exciting and maybe unique, based on values such as partnership, opportunism, backing individuals not structures, organic growth and community ownership."

The Centre has discerned, nurtured, and called for the "great reserves of energy and ability in the local community" through its integrated, holistic approach that is attracting national attention—and now funding. It has been successful in developing partnerships not only with the local people, but also with government and industry and with the academic and philanthropic communities. As it has sought to develop a broad base of support to underwrite its programs and make them less vulnerable, the Centre has also been challenged by "the danger of individual funders withdrawing precisely because of the broad base, and the time needed to administer, monitor and report to many different funders."

The Centre has recognized that "in communities such as Bromley by Bow where resources rarely meet the level of need, there is an interplay between those who traditionally control change and those who receive it. Health is right at the heart of this interplay because the ability to create positive change is dependent on a broad sense of well being and confidence." The new Health Centre continues to model its belief that people need to "engage in a process of transformation which enables people to own their own bodies and the services which assist them, not just be participants in a system set up for them and controlled by someone else."

Christ House

1717 Columbia Road, NW
Washington, D.C. 20009
Telephone: (202) 328-1100; fax: (202) 232-4972
Contact: Dr. Janelle Goetcheus, Medical Director; Scott Gunn,
  Administrative Director

Mission and Activities. Christ House (CH) provides twenty-four-hour, direct health care for about 250 sick, homeless men per year and assistance in addressing critical issues to break the cycle of homelessness. The thirty-four-bed medical facility allows homeless patients to stay as long as their illness requires, getting plenty of rest, nutritious meals, medical care, and social services. "If I were President of the United States," says one patient, "I couldn't get any better treatment than I do at Christ House." In addition, arrangements are made for an average of ten patients per day to visit specialists and receive hospital and clinic care.

What makes the ministry unique is that many of the staff members live at Christ House with their families, building a community of empathy and friendship with those who are hurting in body and spirit. "The thread holding the whole operation together is a carefully nurtured sense of community among staff and patients."

CH also provides office space for Unity Health Care, Inc. (formerly the Health Care for the Homeless Project), a pilot program that makes Christ House the national base for the country's outreach efforts to the homeless. The Unity Clinic is one of twelve in the District of Columbia.

Sponsor. Church of the Saviour, 2025 Massachusetts Avenue, NW, Washington, D.C., which consists of nine small faith communities totaling 130 members. From it have sprung Jubilee Ministries (of which Christ House is a part) and dozens of other mission projects.

Governance. Self-perpetuating board of directors of Christ House and Kairos House professional staff.

Financial Support. CH is supported by more than 6,500 individuals, churches, businesses, associations, corporations, and foundations. Total budget for 1998 was $2,049,576. Forty percent of the funding comes from a homeless service grant from the Department of Housing and Urban Development (HUD).

Composition of Staff. There are 42 staff: 12 administrative, 16 health care, 2 social services, 1 pastoral care, 7 food services, and 4 maintenance. There are also 250 volunteers per month plus 7 full-time, year-long volunteers who provide $282,566 in labor costs.

Persons Served. Homeless, sick men in metropolitan Washington, D.C.

Types of Services. *Liturgical.* Residents gather Thursday and Sunday for worship led by Allen Goetcheus, a Methodist pastor, in the chapel or prayer room. A Bible study, "Bread of Life," and a group on Spirituality Today also meet weekly led by Sister Marcella Jordan.

Educational. Daily educational activities such as tutoring, art, and poetry workshops are offered to foster self-esteem and build social skills.

Support/Advocacy. Alcoholic Anonymous meetings are arranged since about half of the patients have serious alcohol problems. Alternative housing arrangements are found for more than 65 percent of patients when they are discharged from Christ House; Kairos House, also part of Jubilee Ministries, has thirty-seven apartments for independent living, though many of Christ House residents can never live independently. To represent the needs of the homeless for health care, including mental health services, the staff becomes involved in public policy advocacy.

Direct Health Services. Patients spend an average of thirty-nine days at Christ House. Each guest receives loving, excellent care from a team that includes a physician, a nurse, a social worker, and a volunteer coordinator. The services of a psychiatrist are also available for those with mental illness in addition to their physical ailments. This 20,000-square-foot facility has meeting rooms, a dining hall, patient rooms with nurses' station, a social room, and staff apartments.

Background and History. As reporters for the Christian monthly *Sojourners* and for *Physician* magazine tell the story, Janelle Goetcheus, a family physician, and her husband, Allen, a Methodist minister, were preparing in 1975 to leave their home in Indiana to be missionaries in Pakistan. Waiting for their visas, they visited Washington, D.C., and saw that they did not have to go overseas to help the poor. "It was my first exposure to the terrible conditions some people live in," Janelle told *Physician* magazine. "I saw those people, and the needs struck me. I knew I wanted to help." The Goetcheuses ended up staying in Washington, D.C., and in 1979, Janelle founded Columbia Road Health Services, an inner-city health clinic and ministry of the ecumenical Church of the Saviour. Daily she walked by an abandoned, trash-filled four-story building near the clinic. Homeless people slept out on its front steps, and in bitterly cold weather they might go inside to sleep, starting fires to keep warm. Janelle prayed that one day this abandoned building might be put to use for the homeless. "Her resolve was strengthened when a man she had seen at the clinic one snowy afternoon was found frozen to death in a telephone booth the next day."

Overcoming Obstacles and Challenges. The initial obstacle to starting Christ House "was no money for such a place where the homeless sick could rest and recover, a temporary home for those too sick to be on the streets but not sick enough to be in a hospital. The task of creating such a home seemed overwhelming. But Janelle shared her vision with Gordon Cosby, pastor of Church of the Saviour. He turned to a woman he knew, who gave $2.5 million for the purchase of the abandoned building, renovation costs, and the first months of operation. The first patient walked through the doors of Christ House on Christmas Eve in 1985." Both Janelle and her husband—who serves as pastor to the community at Christ House—not only work but also live with other staff and their families at Christ House. The clinic has opened its doors to more than three thousand of the city's homeless men since the first patient walked inside more than two decades ago.

The ongoing challenges of this ministry are financial, that is, raising sufficient funds as well as meeting the overwhelming health and social needs of the homeless. When Gunn and Goetcheus were asked how they avoided burnout, they replied, "A disciplined prayer life, a strong sense of God's call, and the community of other staff."

Church Health Center of Memphis, Inc.

1210 Peabody Avenue
Memphis, Tennessee 38104-4570
Telephone: (901) 272-0003; fax: (901) 272-7179
Contact: Rev. G. Scott Morris, M.D., Executive Director; Jean
   Campbell, Director

Mission and Activities. The Church Health Center (CHC) is a cooperative effort by 175 Memphis churches that have banded together across denominational lines to build a health ministry that has strongly impacted their community. It seeks to reclaim the biblical and historical commitment of the church to care for the poor and respond to God's calling to heal and teach. The Center annually records about 30,000 patient visits and has served more than 28,000 individual patients of the city's low-income uninsured working people with support from all of the city's major hospitals. Located in downtown Memphis, the Center is unique in that its founder and chief physician, G. Scott Morris, is also an ordained United Methodist pastor. He ministers to his own medical and support staff by supporting them in their faith journeys and providing pastoral care.

"The Center provides all the health care services offered by a family physician's office, plus the benefit of extended services to treat the whole person—body, mind and spirit. Services include medical, dental and optometry care as well as pastoral counseling and preventive health education." While maintaining its primary health care services, the CHC is broadening its base as an educational and resource organization for preventive health care.

Sponsors. More than 175 Memphis worshiping communities ranging from evangelical to liberal, from Protestant and Roman Catholic to Jewish.

Governance. The board of directors is composed of twenty-seven members of the Memphis community who also have been long-time supporters and volunteers of the Center. Nine of the board members are medical professionals, and five are clergy from local churches. As a primary health care provider, the CHC is also governed by federal and state regulatory authorities including the Clinical Laboratory Improvements Act, the Tennessee Department of Radiological Health, and the Tennessee Occupational Safety and Health Act.

Financial Support. The CHC operating budget is about $3 million. Medical costs account for about 58 percent of the expenditures. Patients pay fees on a sliding scale depending upon their ability to pay. Income received from patients covers about one-third of the medical and dental operating costs, and the other two-thirds are covered by donations— mainly from sponsoring church members. A development board, which is separate from the board of directors, is responsible for fund-raising.

Composition of Staff. Starting with a staff of five in 1987, the CHC now employs sixty people. The senior staff consists of the executive director, director, clinic administrator, business administrator, and preventive health director. The medical staff consists of five board-certified physicians and six nurses. They are supported by medical assistants and office staff.

Volunteers. Currently about 100 primary care physicians and 65 dentists donate their time at CHC once a month. Many of them are members of local congregations. In addition, Center patients may be referred to approximately 300 volunteer specialists such as cardiologists and gynecologists; 600 nonmedical volunteers handle a variety of tasks from providing clerical support to organizing donated medicine. By completing dense and complicated paperwork, for example, volunteers have obtained $12,000 worth of donated medicine a month for patients, contributing the equivalent of $300,000 annually through their efforts. CHC is able to attract volunteers because it does not abuse their time. It has a firm policy of refusing to let any health care volunteer work more than once a month or to call a specialist more than twice a month.

Persons Served. The low-income uninsured working people of Memphis who cannot afford to pay the premiums for medical insurance but do not qualify for Medicaid.

Types of Services. *Liturgical.* The founder and chief physician is also an ordained minister and so performs liturgical functions as needed by the staff.

Educational. CHC hopes to change the way medicine is practiced with its thrust toward preventive care through the Hope and Healing Center established in 1999. Its goal is to make health care more than prescribing pills and performing surgery. The $6 million to renovate the 80,000-square-foot sanctuary has already been pledged. The Hope and Healing Center will have a therapeutic pool and exercise equipment, like most gyms, and will also have a staff on hand to counsel both individuals and area congregations on how to prepare healthy, low-fat meals and develop healthy lifestyles. The facility will function as a type of inner-city health facility for the working poor on the premise that two-thirds of the cases treated at the clinic could have been avoided with lifestyle changes. "Prescriptions for health," to promote wellness through diet and exercise, will be "filled" at the Hope and Healing Center (the University of Tennessee Department of Preventive Medicine is currently working closely with the Center staff to determine whether lifestyle changes are taken more seriously by patients when they are actually prescribed in writing rather than offered as general advice by a doctor).

Dr. Morris's vision is for doctors to start writing prescriptions for health, a practice he currently follows at CHC's clinic. Just as doctors now use protocols to help them diagnose prescriptions for the sick, so new protocols can be developed for prescriptions that keep people healthy. Low-impact exercise, weight loss, smoking cessation—these are the prescriptions that need to be filled to cure diabetes, arthritis, and heart failure. The question is where? A doctor will not write a prescription unless it can be filled. The Center sees the Hope and Healing Center as such a location. Churches practicing health ministries will be other places where people can fill their prescriptions.

"When you walk into a church today it's normal to see a music program, Christian education, and adult Bible study," says Julia Hicks, a member of the Hope and Healing staff. "But the churches are killing us with their potluck suppers as they are saving our souls. In the future there will also be a smoking cessation class, an arthritis recovery class, stretching and strength building." The beauty of health ministry programs is not only their sound theological basis but also their low cost. "What we're finding is that hardly any of this preventive health is expensive," says Hicks.

Support/Advocacy. The Center's patients often are referred to pastoral counselors when the doctor determines that the chest pain they are complaining about is really a broken heart. Besides psychological and spiritual support, the Center is trying to address the sociopolitical causes of sickness through its work with elementary school children in a low-income area of the city. Its pilot project is examining the systemic causes of ill health from unemployment, domestic violence, crime, drugs, dilapidated housing, and the pressures of single parenthood. All of these conditions adversely affect the 1,100 students at Caldwell Elementary School, whose principal asked the Center staff for help because her students were frequently out sick from school. Twenty-five area churches have "adopted" the school to support the Center's effort to create an atmosphere that elevates the health of the children. As a first step a health curriculum is being implemented through the use of drama, and a local ballet company is introducing creative body movement to the children. In addition, the Center has developed the MEMPHIS Plan, "a health care plan for uninsured, near-minimum-wage workers."

Direct Health Services. At the Center's medical clinic, patients pay what they are able or a minimum of $10 a visit for medical care, $20 for an optometry exam and a pair of eyeglasses. The Center also operates a walk-in clinic for people with broken bones, lacerations, or the flu who need immediate attention and have been turned away by emergency rooms.

Background and History. CHC embodies the vision of Scott Morris, a Yale Divinity School and medical school graduate who seeks to fulfill "the biblical command of caring for the poor and the sick." "I think of myself as a pastor who acquired a particular skill," he says with typical modesty. From the beginning Morris believed that health care should be affordable to the working poor and that the patient should pay for medical services.

Overcoming Obstacles and Challenges. Dr. Morris's number one obstacle when he arrived in Memphis in 1987 to pursue his dream was that he did not know anyone. He was fortunate to begin work as an associate pastor at St. John's United Methodist Church where he still teaches Sunday school. The senior pastor, Frank McRae, was one of the best-connected men in Memphis after nineteen years in ministry. Reverend McRae introduced Morris to the African American community, which surrounded his parish and now accounts for about 70 percent of CHC's patients.

Not only did Reverend McRae have connections, but he also had a broad enough view not to claim ownership of the health ministry Morris wanted to start. He opened the idea up and "brought to the rich and poor in the faith community a message about the opportunity to heal." Known as a liberal, McRae approached one of the most conservative evangelical pastors in town and asked him for help to start the Center. The pastor happened to have a wealthy family in his congregation who wanted to contribute to a medical healing project. The family gave $120,000 to renovate a building for the Center.

Dr. Morris then approached Methodist Health Care Systems for operating funds through its health and welfare ministries committee. The hospital was not initially enthusiastic. There was a major concern that staff physicians at the hospital would see the Center as competition. But Morris persevered. After internal debate in committee meetings, the hospital agreed to give $100,000 and has remained a loyal supporter. Then the Jewish-based Plough Foundation provided $100,000 for the first year of operation.

From the beginning the sources of funding for the Center were diverse and ecumenical, setting the stage for 175 other churches to climb aboard the effort because it was open to everyone. Most churches did not want to create something insular. "We avoided that," notes Butch Odom, the Center's business administrator, who attributes the Center's success to its broad base and generous initial funding that have generally allowed the Center to operate at a surplus over the years.

The funds have filtered in, Center staff say, because money follows ideas, and people give to people. All agree that Morris woke up the faith community to the real issues. "They got behind him," remembers Jean Campbell, who turned Morris down twice before she eventually agreed to assume her current responsibilities as the Center director because of Morris's persistence. The success of the Church Health Center has been so impressive that people have traveled from as far away as China and India to witness the ministry and its charismatic doctor.

Glide Memorial Methodist Church

Addiction Recovery Program
330 Ellis Street
San Francisco, California 94102
Telephone: (415) 771-6300; fax: (415) 921-6951
Contact: Rev. Cecil Williams, Senior Pastor; Sally Anderson, Public
 Relations

Mission and Activities. Glide Memorial is a six-story church in the Tenderloin District of San Francisco. It reaches out to its immediate community of drug pushers and users, prostitutes and pimps and people who felt beyond hope and recovery but come through the doors of Glide's Fellowship Hall and find new life. Reverend Williams's vision of a one-stop church that meets all the congregation's spiritual, physical, emotional, and socioeconomic needs enhances the process of recovery and ensures a much higher rate of success. In fact, Glide's statistics show a 70 to 80 percent success rate for people staying in recovery and establishing careers, which far exceeds the rate of other programs. The Addiction Recovery Program is the center of its ministry.

The recovery "workshops" Glide has developed are not typical twelve-step meetings. One of the distinguishing features is the use of loving confrontation. "Get your act together and change your life" is the message delivered in no uncertain terms, on the one hand, and acceptance if you don't, on the other. "Unconditional love and support for all" is the phrase most often heard. The people who gather for the addiction recovery workshops listen to each other's stories. They respond out of their own lives of addiction and recovery and challenge people to get serious about what they are doing. "Are you ready?" is the main question. People in recovery themselves become counselors. These new counselors often go on to college to get counseling degrees and leave the Glide program to work in other well-established community-based programs. So the benefit of going through the Glide program is not only recovery but becoming equipped to work outside the church, hence, starting a new life.

Sponsors. Glide Memorial Methodist Church, city organizations and agencies.

Governance. A board of directors.

Financial Support. Grassroots fund-raising efforts in the community as well as banquets with the mayor and other dignitaries who pay five hundred dollars a plate to support the church; private and government funding.

Composition of Staff. The pastor who directs the overall program as well as counselors (many of whom are recovering addicts) and individual staff for each one of the auxiliary programs.

Persons Served. Residents of the Tenderloin District, San Francisco, especially drug pushers, users, prostitutes, pimps, and people who are beyond hope and recovery. In addition, local celebrities, movie stars, and wealthy people who may be battling addiction or looking for a spiritual home, and visitors to the church.

Types of Services. *Liturgical.* Sunday morning worship at Glide rocks with a seventy-five-member choir, drums, trumpet, organ, piano, and a choreographer/signer. Graduates from the church's recovery program share their testimonies of recovery during the service. For those walking into the church for the first time, this becomes a powerful witness about how they can change.

While Glide ministers to the surrounding Tenderloin community, it is a church that includes gay and straight, rich and poor, believers and non-believers—a rainbow coalition of people from all economic, racial, and social classes. They come together in a celebration that is very reminiscent of a black Baptist church, even though it is Methodist. So vibrant is worship that tourists to San Francisco from all over the world come for the experience. The people line up outside the church to sit in the balcony and the main sanctuary called Freedom Hall.

Educational. Job skills and career counseling programs are offered through a three-week workshop for people to learn how to do interviews, fill out job application forms, and discover their skills and how to present them. Computer skills, employment assistance programs, addiction prevention materials—these and other approaches equip those who have been helpless and hopeless to start a new life.

Support/Advocacy. Trust is a big part of the Addiction Recovery Program at Glide; Williams still continues to nurture the caring atmosphere that built his church by walking around the six floors of Glide to talk with the people. His office is on the first floor where he is available and accessible to people who walk in off the street.

By witnessing to the power of God to change lives, the church has become an advocate for those whom society has rejected. The counseling and recovery groups are part of the ongoing support of the most needy.

Direct Health Services. There is a level of sophistication to Glide's Addiction Recovery Program not typically found in church-based ministries. Church staff establish case management reports on the people in recovery and do follow-up. In addition to the support groups open to anyone, Glide offers a Generation follow-up program of recovery in which participants sign a seventeen-week contract that may be court mandated. Glide is recognized by the San Francisco court system for its effective work following initial recovery. Graduates of the program wear buttons with the legend, "I am a Generation Graduate"; there are now about twenty-eight generations.

The open addiction recovery meetings begin with a song printed on sheets for everyone to sing. People sign in, another departure from twelve-step programs where anonymity is stressed. Then each person briefly tells his or her story. A volunteer counselor might break in after a person shares and say, "Okay, we've heard your story. Now are you really going to commit to change, or is this just kind of something you're thinking about? How serious are you?" And the counselor might continue with this line of conversation for about fifteen minutes. Sometimes an assistant counselor might stay all day with an addict—those I met hungered for a friend and sympathetic ear.

The church serves hot meals to long lines of hundreds of homeless and destitute people every day of the week during the morning, noon, and evening hours. People may come to Glide to get a free meal; however, this may be the first step toward a sense of hope and recovery in their lives. Glide is building a primary health care clinic and a high-rise building next to the church, which will offer housing and apartments for single men, women, or families who have been homeless. There will be no limit to the time they can stay.

Background and History. The vision for the ministry at Glide stems from Rev. Cecil Williams, who has been laboring in the Tenderloin District neighborhood for the past thirty years. He started Glide with a near-empty church that had no connection to the neighborhood. As he walked the blocks that surrounded the church and saw the hopelessness and addictive cycle of the local people's lives, he vowed the church would do something.

Overcoming Obstacles and Challenges. As Glide's greatest asset, Williams is also the church's greatest liability since there is a danger that the program will die when such a charismatic leader departs. Recognizing this, Williams currently is training his successor, who will be an essential piece to the continuity of the Glide program.

In addition, Williams has written of his own struggle with addictive behavior in terms of workaholism and codependency—trying to be all things to all people—a dilemma most clergy can relate to in their congregational ministry. He found that he needed to give up believing he had to "be there" in order to make things happen; he needed to let go of his own sense of importance to regain healthy boundaries for himself and thereby become a better minister to others. He recognized he could not solve people's problems for them. They had to solve them for themselves.

MAP (Medical Assistance Programs) International

2200 Glynco Parkway, P.O. Box 215000
Brunswick, Georgia 31521
Telephone: (800) 225-8550; fax: (912) 265-6170
E-mail: mapus@map.org; Web site: <http://www.map.org>
Contact: Paul Thompson, President and Chief Executive Officer

Mission and Activities. "MAP International is a Christian relief and development non-profit organization which provides medicine and hospital supplies in more than 100 countries to meet long-term health needs and to aid in disaster relief in the world's poorest communities." It partners in the provision of essential medicines, prevention and eradication of disease, and the promotion of community health development. Its head-quarters are in Brunswick, Georgia, in a 45,000-square-foot facility, of which 35,000 square feet function as a medical distribution warehouse. International offices are in Nairobi, Kenya; Quito, Ecuador; Chilimarca, Bolivia; and Abidjan, Ivory Coast.

Sponsors. "A not-for-profit Christian global health organization, MAP is supported by an international network of churches, individuals, corporations and foundations."

Governance. MAP has a thirteen-member board of directors as well as five officers of the board, including the chairman, vice chairman, secretary, treasurer, and president. A nonvoting board of governors advises the board and the president/CEO.

Financial Support. Revenue of more than $100 million annually is primarily from in-kind contributions from health care companies. During the 1996–97 fiscal year MAP received $141 million in donated medicine. Cash donations are received from churches, individuals, and foundations.

Composition of Staff. A twelve-member global leadership team directs the efforts of a worldwide staff of about one hundred, approximately fifty of whom are based in the United States. There are four permanent volunteers on site in Brunswick, Georgia. Twice a month, approximately sixty community volunteers come to the headquarters warehouse to pack medicines for short-term projects.

In addition, a number of doctors and health professionals who are not affiliated with MAP utilize its services to procure medicines to take with them on their own volunteer efforts overseas. For a $375 handling fee, MAP provides them with a "physician's travel pack," which typically contains about $5,000 worth of medicine.

Persons Served. The world's poorest communities, including those in Latin America, Africa, India, and the Commonwealth of Independent States (CIS).

Types of Services. *Educational.* MAP is training more than five hundred village health promoters and other grassroots leaders in Latin America and Africa about wholistic health (social, spiritual, emotional, and cultural needs of communities); educating church leaders on the issue of AIDS; translating AIDS manuals into native languages; and holding workshops for women regarding HIV/AIDS and the church. In addition, "MAP has sponsored the training of more than 1,700 senior medical students from the U.S. and Canada in overseas mission hospitals in order to encourage their commitment to health care in the developing world."

Support/Advocacy. Promotion of wholistic health includes clergy workshops on peace and reconciliation in war-torn countries.

Direct Health Services. MAP annually distributes approximately $100 million worth of medicine and medical supplies, some of which it receives through donations from seventy-two leading U.S. health care companies. "These medicines are distributed to hospitals, clinics, agencies and relief centers in 100 countries.

"MAP responds to emergencies caused by war and natural disasters in places like Bosnia, Burundi, Uganda, Tanzania, Rwanda, Ecuador and the United States; and assesses the needs of Christian hospitals, clinics and dispensaries worldwide to see how MAP and other agencies can serve them."

Background and History. "Founded in 1954 as the Medical Assistance Programs of the Christian Medical Society, MAP first began providing donated medicines to health care workers traveling into the developing world to assist hospitals and clinics serving the poor." The effort was started by Dr. Raymond Knighton, a physician whose own medical trips made him see the great lack of medicines in the developing world. He contacted pharmaceutical companies whose donated medicines soon filled his garage and paved the way for MAP. Distribution of medicines proceeded at such a high volume over the years that in 1985 MAP relocated to Brunswick, Georgia, because it was midway between the deep-water shipping ports of Savannah, Georgia, and Jacksonville, Florida. "Over the past four decades MAP has strengthened and expanded its work to meet the health needs of the whole person—physical, social and spiritual, with its major programs in the promotion of community health development, the provision of essential medicines and medical supplies and the prevention and eradication of disease."

Overcoming Challenges and Obstacles. When one considers that more than two billion people lack essential medicine and 75 percent of illnesses in young children in developing countries are preventable, one of the greatest challenges MAP experiences is meeting people at their point of need with appropriate and timely medicines and services. MAP recently supplied Hepatitis A vaccine for a countrywide vaccination campaign in Ecuador, distributed more than 53,000 doses of flu vaccine to the poor at dozens of clinics throughout the United States, and more than one million doses of polio vaccine in Africa and Latin America. Through MAP, thousands of children received a vaccination for a disease that is virtually unknown in the United States.

One of the greatest long-term challenges in the provision of services is enabling people to help themselves. This has been a primary focus of MAP International's work. MAP's production of indigenous, culturally relevant HIV/AIDS-related materials and prevention programs have changed countless lives in Africa, Asia, Latin America, and the United States. The self-sustaining, community-based health training centers in Latin America have given hands-on training to more than 220 people from both urban and rural areas, providing lasting change and a hope for the future.

CONCLUSION

As was stated throughout this book, now is the fullness of time for men and women of faith, as individuals and as a community, to respond to Christ's call to heal. This is the moment for the church to truly become *the healing church*, developing new methods and programs to meet the needs of God's people.

Having read the stories of the wonderful health ministry programs in the United States and the United Kingdom and several other countries, may you, the reader, go forth to start new programs or feel energized to continue and expand your current one. May God who calls us, who equips us, and who heals us empower us for this ministry—to heed the cries of the sick and suffering, whether of body, mind, or spirit, and to preach and live the liberating word of Jesus Christ.

Notes

1. THE CHURCH'S HISTORIC ROLE IN HEALTH AND HEALING

1. See Abigail Rian Evans, *Redeeming Marketplace Medicine: A Theology of Health Care* (Cleveland: The Pilgrim Press, 1999).

2. Ronald Numbers and Darrel Amundsen, eds., *Caring and Curing: Health and Medicine in the Western Religious Tradition* (New York: Macmillan, 1986); Lauren E. Sullivan, ed., *Healing and Restoration: Health and Medicine in the World's Religious Tradition* (Baltimore: Johns Hopkins University Press, 1989).

3. Charles Gusmer, *The Ministry of Healing in the Church of England as Ecumenical-Liturgical Study*, the Alcuin Club Collections, no. 56 (London: Heron and Co., 1974), 26. Gusmer relies on article 6 of the *Archbishop's Report, 1958* to make this argument based on the sufficiency of Scripture.

4. Evelyn Frost, *Christian Healing: A Consideration of the Place of Spiritual Healing in the Church of Today in the Light of the Doctrine and Practice of the Ante-Nicene Church* (London: A. R. Mowbray & Co., 1940), 19.

5. See Evans, *Redeeming Marketplace Medicine*, for an extensive discussion of Christ's healing ministry.

6. Frost, *Christian Healing*, 57.

7. Morris Maddocks, *The Christian Healing Ministry* (London: SPCK, 1981), 79. Maddocks cites Acts 9:40–42, the raising of Tabitha.

8. Ibid., 85.

9. Ibid.

10. James H. Charlesworth, professor of New Testament at Princeton Theological Seminary, Princeton, New Jersey, provided the information on the *zeqenim*.

11. Leuven Institute lectures, Belgium, summer 1997, 15.

12. Maddocks, *The Christian Healing Ministry*, 117.

13. Leuven Institute lectures, 15.

14. Maddocks, *The Christian Healing Ministry*, 118.

15. Gusmer, *The Ministry of Healing*, 32.

16. John Crowlesmith, "Non-Medical Healing from the Age of the Fathers to the Evangelical Revival," in *Religion and Medicine*, ed. John Crowlesmith (London: Epworth Press, 1962), 20.

17. Ignatius, "Letter to the Ephesians," paragraph 10, in *Early Christian Fathers*, ed. Cyril C. Richardson (New York: Touchstone, 1996), 91.

18. Ignatius, "Letter to the Magnesians," para. 13, in *Early Christian Fathers*, 97.

19. James S. Jeffers, *Conflict at Rome: Social Order and Hierarchy in Early Christianity* (Minneapolis: Fortress Press, 1991), 107–12.

20. Hermas, "III Hermas: Similitudes," 5.59, in *The Lost Books of the Bible* (New York: Alpha Publishing Company, 1926), 235.

21. Cyprian, "To the Lapsed," chapter 26, in *St. Cyprian: The Lapsed; The Unity of the Catholic Church*, translated and annotated by Maurice Bévenot, Ancient Christian Writers series, no. 25 (Westminster, Md.: Newman Press, 1957), 35.

22. Crowlesmith, "Non-Medical Healing," 20.

23. Ibid.

24. Ibid.

25. Justin Martyr, "Dialogue w/ Trypho," 39, in *The Ante-Nicene Fathers: Translations of the Writings of the Fathers Down to AD 325*, vol. 1, ed. Alexander Roberts and James Donaldson (Christian Classics Ethereal Library, on-line <www.ccel.wheaton.edu>).

26. Irenaeus, "Against Heresies," 2.31.2, in *The Ante-Nicene Fathers: Translations of the Writings of the Fathers Down to AD 325*, vol. 1.

27. Gusmer, *The Ministry of Healing*, 39.

28. Crowlesmith, "Non-Medical Healing," 20.

29. R. J. S. Barrett-Lennard, *The Sacramentary of Sarapion of Thumis: A Text for Students, with Introduction, Translation, and Commentary* (Bramcote, Eng.: Grove Books Limited, 1993), 18.

30. Paul Bradshaw, ed., *The Canons of Hippolytus* (Bramcote, Eng.: Grove Books Limited, 1987), canons 5, 21, 24, pp. 14, 26, 27.

31. Ibid., canon 8, p. 16.

32. Ibid., canons 19 and 25, pp. 21, 28.

33. Theophilus of Antioch, "To Autolycus," 26, in *The Ante-Nicene Fathers: Translations of the Writings of the Fathers Down to AD 325*, vol. 2.

34. Tertullian, "To Scapula," 4, and Tertullian, "Apology," 32, in *The Ante-Nicene Fathers: Translations of the Writings of the Fathers Down to AD 325*, vol. 3.

35. Bradshaw, *The Canons of Hippolytus*, canon 19, p. 21.

36. St. Augustine, *Concerning the City of God Against the Pagans*, 22.8, trans. Henry Bettenson (Harmondsworth, Eng.: Penguin Books, 1972), 1033–47.

37. Stephen Pattison, *Alive and Kicking* (London: SCM Press, 1993), 47.

38. Ibid., 48.

39. Of course, it was during this period that debates about consubstantiation and transubstantiation were raging. See further J. N. D. Kelly, *Early Christian Doctrines*, rev. ed. (San Francisco: Harper & Row, 1978), 440–55.

40. Leuven Institute lectures, 18.

41. Ibid.

42. James McGilvray, *The Quest for Health and Wholeness* (Tubingen: German Institute for Medical Missions, 1981), 2.

43. Phyllis Garlick, *The Wholeness of Man: A Study in the History of Healing* (London: Highway Press, 1943), 102.

44. Gusmer, *The Ministry of Healing*, 38.

45. Garlick, *The Wholeness of Man*, 102.

46. McGilvray, *The Quest for Health and Wholeness*, 3.

47. Garlick, *The Wholeness of Man*, 102.

48. H. Fielding Garrison, *History of Medicine* (London, 1929), quoted in Garlick, *The Wholeness of Man*, 102–3.

49. Garlick, *The Wholeness of Man*, 103.

50. Ibid., 103–4.

51. Ibid., 104.

52. McGilvray, *The Quest for Health and Wholeness*, 3.

53. St. Mary of Bethlehem was the first hospital for the mentally ill. Over time the name was shortened to Beddelem, later to Bedlem, and became a new English word to indicate the destructiveness of disease—bedlam.

54. Darrel W. Amundsen and Gary B. Ferngren, "The Early Christian Tradition," in *Caring and Curing*, 58; Darrel W. Amundsen, "The Medieval Catholic Tradition," in *Caring and Curing*, 84–85.

55. Gusmer, *The Ministry of Healing*, 32.

56. Leuven Institute lectures, 22.

57. Amundsen, "The Medieval Catholic Tradition," 74.

58. Ibid., 80.

59. Frederick Behrends, ed. and trans., "Letter 71, Archbishop H[ugh] of Tours, to Bishop H[ubert] of Angers, before 10 June 1023," in *The Letters and Poems of Fulbert of Chartres* (Oxford: Clarendon Press, 1976), 121.

60. Amundsen, "The Medieval Catholic Tradition," 75.

61. Stephen Parsons, *The Challenge of Christian Healing* (London: SPCK, 1981), 151.

62. Thomas Aquinas, *Summa Theologiae*, Supplement Question 30, Article 1, trans. Fathers of the English Dominican Province (Christian Classics Ethereal Library, on-line <www.ccel.wheaton.edu>).

63. Rev. H. J. Schroeder, trans., *The Canons and Decrees of the Council of Trent*, 13.8 (Rockford, Ill.: Tan Books and Publishers, 1978), 78. See further Stanley Samuel Harakas, "The Eastern Orthodox Tradition," in *Caring and Curing*, 151 ff. It is instructive to note, however, that generally during the early Byzantine period (324–700 c.e.) there was no essential conflict in Eastern Christian theology between science and philosophy and affirmations of faith. There was a convergence of the spirit of philanthropy and appreciation of medicine. Many well-known and innovative physicians such as St. John Chrysostom (345–407 c.e.), patriarch of Constantinople, established hospitals in the Byzantine capital staffed by clergy as directors and hired doctors, cooks, attendants, and nurses. However, in the sixth and seventh centuries the medical profession lost its standing, and hagiography waged a war against secular physicians, which lasted until the twelfth century.

64. Schroeder, *The Canons and Decrees of the Council of Trent*, 14.3, 90–91. Penance preceded unction with parts of contrition, confession, and satisfaction.

65. Ibid., 14.9, 99.

66. J. R. Pridie, *The Church's Ministry of Healing* (1926), 85–86, quoted in Gusmer, *The Ministry of Healing*, 48.

67. Schroeder, *The Canons and Decrees of the Council of Trent*, 14.3, 101.

68. Ibid., 14.2, 100.

69. John Calvin, *Institutes of the Christian Religion*, 2 vols., ed. John T. McNeill, trans. Ford Lewis Battle (Philadelphia: Westminster Press, 1960), 1:706.

70. Ibid., 1:35–39.

71. C. W. Baird, *Eutaxia, or the Presbyterian Liturgies: Historical Sketches* (New York: M. W. Dodd, Publishers, 1855), 122.

72. Richard Baxter, "Directions for the Sick," in *The Practical Works of Richard Baxter*, 4 vols. (London: Arthur Hall and Co., 1854), 1:522–47.

73. Ibid., 1:534.

74. Ibid., 1:522–47.

75. David Gregg, ed., *Ministry to the Sick: An Introduction*, Grove Worship Series no. 58 (Bramcote, Eng.: Grove Books, 1978), 12.

76. Colin Buchanan and David Wheaton, *Liturgy for the Sick: The New Church of England Services*, Grove Worship Series no. 84 (Bramcote, Eng.: Grove Books, 1983), 18.

77. Ibid., 3.

78. Smylie, "The Reformed Tradition," 208; Marvin R. O'Connell, "The Roman Catholic Tradition Since 1545," in *Caring and Curing*, 135. It should be noted, however, the Catholic Counter Reformation burst forth with fresh communities of women such as the Ursulines to serve the sick in the sixteenth century, and produced the highly influential Sisters of Charity of St. Vincent de Paul in the seventeenth century.

79. Garlick, *The Wholeness of Man*, 105–6.

80. Ibid., 106.

81. In the twentieth century these social concerns led to active engagement in health care reform on all fronts. See chapter 6 for discussion of health care reform.

82. Crowlesmith, "Non-Medical Healing," 26.

83. Morton Kelsey, *Healing and Christianity* (New York: Harper & Row, 1973), quoted in Parsons, *The Challenge of Christian Healing*, 148–49. Parsons also argues that most Protestant theologians were opposed to the healing ministry of the church and cites Barth as an example because he says so little about it in his *Church Dogmatics*.

84. Garlick, *The Wholeness of Man*, 120.

85. Ibid., 48.

86. Ibid.

87. Ibid., 63.

88. Ibid., 129.

89. Ibid., 66.

90. Ibid., 133.

91. Kristin Gleeson, *Healers Abroad: Presbyterian Women Physicians in the Foreign Mission Field* (Temple University, May 1996), 167.

92. Ibid., 180.

93. Robert Ellis, Associate for Program Development and Resourcing, International Health Ministries Office of Worldwide Ministries, Division of Presbyterian Church USA, Louisville, Kentucky, telephone interview by Jane Ferguson, research assistant, 14 November 1996.

94. Of course, there were many exceptions to this with the work of the Christian Medical Commission of the World Council of Churches, innovative community-based health education programs, as well as those by the PCUSA with Dr. John Sibley in Korea in the 1960s and 1970s, and other such innovators.

95. Pattison, *Alive and Kicking*, 69 ff. See also pages 56–58 of my book for a critique of faith healers.

96. Frost, *Christian Healing*, 183.

97. Denis Duncan, *Pastoral Care and Ethical Issues* (Edinburgh: Saint Andrew Press, 1988).

98. Buchanan and Wheaton, *Liturgy for the Sick*, 18–19.

99. Gusmer, *The Ministry of Healing*, 10 ff.

100. Ibid., 10–12.

101. Maddocks, *The Christian Healing Ministry*, 101.

102. Morris Maddocks, *Journey to Wholeness* (London: SPCK, 1986), 79.

103. Gusmer, *The Ministry of Healing*, 14.

104. Ibid., 56 ff., infers these three types but they are not explicit in the text.

105. Maddocks, *The Christian Healing Ministry*, 120.

106. Purcell Fox, *The Church's Ministry of Healing* (London: Longmans, 1959), 59.

107. Gusmer, *The Ministry of Healing*, 9.

108. Ibid., 10.

109. Lambeth Conference proceedings, quoted by Maddocks, *The Christian Healing Ministry*, 113–14.

110. Maddocks, *Journey to Wholeness*, 223–24.

111. Gusmer, *The Ministry of Healing*, 22.

112. See the discussion on "odic" force in chapter 2.

113. Maddocks, *The Christian Healing Ministry*, 107–8.

114. Ibid., 109.

115. Pattison, *Alive and Kicking*, 56–57.

116. Garlick, *The Wholeness of Man*, 111.

117. J. Wesley, *Primitive Physic, or, An Easy and Natural Method of Curing Most Diseases* (London: G. Paramore, 1792).

118. Garlick, *The Wholeness of Man*, 113.

119. Ibid., 114.

120. Pattison, *Alive and Kicking*, 90. See further Granger Westberg, ed., *Theological Roots of Wholistic Health Care: A Response to the Religious Questions Which Have Been Raised* (Hinsdale, Ill.: Wholistic Health Centers, 1979).

121. Pattison, *Alive and Kicking*, 91.

122. Much more could be said on this issue. See especially Allen Verhey and Stephen Lammers, *Theological Voices in Medical Ethics* (Grand Rapids, Mich.: Eerdmans, 1993), and Baruch A. Brody et al., eds., *Theological Developments in Bioethics 1988–1990*, vol. 1 (Boston: Kluwer Academic Publishers, 1991).

123. See Evans, *Redeeming Marketplace Medicine*, for a discussion of the medical model; see also "Global Health and the Limits of Medicine: An Interview with Dave Hilton," *Second Opinion* 18, no. 3 (January 1993): 53–68, for further discussion of health ministries development.

124. Gusmer, *The Ministry of Healing*, 26.

125. Tilda Norberg and Robert Webber, *Stretch Out Your Hand: Exploring Healing Prayer* (Cleveland: United Church Press, 1990), 11.

126. See chapter 8 for a further discussion of parish nursing.

127. "Summary Report: Results, Church Health Survey" (New York: National Council of Churches in the USA, 1991), photocopy, 5.

2. THE FULLNESS OF TIME FOR A NEW HEALTH MINISTRY

1. "Minority Health," *Fastats A to Z*, Statistical Rolodex—Minority Health, <http://www.cdc.gov/nchswww/data/nvsr47-9.pdf> [11 June 1999].

2. United Kingdom, <http://www.odci.gov/cia/publications/factbook/uk.html> [4 November 1998].

3. The Institute for Health & Aging, University of California, San Francisco, *Chronic Care in America: A 21st Century Challenge* (Princeton, N.J.: Robert Wood Johnson Foundation, 1996), 26–27.

4. Leighton Cluff, "Societal Issues Related to Health, Healing, and Health Care" (lecture, n.p., n.d.), 5.

5. D. C. McGilvray, ed., *The Quest for Health: Report of a Study Process* (Cleator Moor, Eng.: Bethwaites Printers, 1979), 15.

6. René Dubos, *The Mirage of Health* (New York: Harper & Row, 1959), 24.

7. "Health in America Tied to Income and Education," press release, U.S. Department of Health and Human Services, <http://www.cdc.gov/nchswww/releases/98news/98news/huspr98.htm> [29 October 1998], 2.

8. A. Sam Warren, "Wholeness in Medicine: Is There a Trinity of Body, Mind, and Spirit?" *Southern Medical Journal,* November 1983.

9. "Family Environment Affects Health of Family Members," press release, National Center for Health Statistics, 1997 Fact Sheets, <http://www.cdc.gov/nchswww/releases/97facts/97sheets/famhealt.htm> [29 October 1998], 2.

10. See Evans, *Redeeming Marketplace Medicine.*

11. The system of fund holders is very controversial right now in the United Kingdom. Doctors, who are assigned to a geographic area from which their patients come, are given a fixed amount of money for all health needs of their patient population and manage and allocate these funds including hospitalization and so forth.

12. Ken Pelletier quoted in John Fitzpatrick, *Create Your Own Health Patterns* (Dublin: Mercier Press, 1980), 78.

13. Nikolas Tinbaergen quoted in ibid., 87.

14. George Howe Colt, "See Me, Feel Me, Touch Me, Heal Me," *Life,* September 1996, 36.

15. Clarissa Kimber, "Building Medical Systems at the Household Level," in *Alternative Therapies: Expanding Options in Health Care,* ed. Rena Gordon, Barbara Niestedt, and Wilbert M. Gesler (New York: Springer, 1996), 149.

16. Ibid., 161.

17. Andrew Weil, *The Marriage of the Sun and Moon* (Boston: Houghton Mifflin, 1980).

18. Colt, "See Me, Feel Me, Touch Me, Heal Me," 46.

19. Ibid., 47.

20. Jeffrey Kluger, "Mr. Natural," *Time,* 12 May 1997, 70. This is the most recent statistic available.

21. *Alternative Medicine: Expanding Medical Horizons—A Report of the National Institutes of Health on Alternative Medical Systems and Practices in the United States* (Washington, D.C.: U.S. Government Printing Office, 1994).

22. Walter Benjamin, review of *Alternative Medicine and American Religious Life,* by Robert C. Fuller, *Christian Century* 107, no. 12 (11 April 1990): 374.

23. Arthur W. Frank, "Where Do I Turn for Healing?" review of *Healing Powers: Alternative Medicine, Spiritual Communities, and the State* by Fred M. Frohock, in *Christian Century* 109, no. 34 (18–25 November 1992): 1063.

24. Colt, "See Me, Feel Me, Touch Me, Heal Me," 38.

25. Benjamin, *Alternative Medicine and American Religious Life,* 374.

26. John T. Chirban, "Healing and Spirituality," in *Health and Faith: Medical, Psychological and Religious Dimensions,* ed. John T. Chirban (Lanham, Md.: University Press of America, 1991), 3–11.

27. "Public Attitudes Toward Massage Study," *Caravan Opinion Research Corporation International,* June 1997, "Trends in Massage Therapy & Complementary Healthcare," Massage Therapy in the United States, <http://www.amtamassage.org/publications/marketresearch.htm> [29 October 1998].

28. *Complementary & Alternative Medicine at NIH* (newsletter) 4, no. 1 (January 1997): 2.

29. Ibid.

30. Colt, "See Me, Feel Me, Touch Me, Heal Me," 36.

31. *Complementary & Alternative Medicine at NIH,* 2.

32. Nancy Scheper-Hughes, *Death without Weeping: The Violence of Everyday Life in Brazil* (Berkeley: University of California Press, 1992), 368–69. A related concept *à míngua* ("to shrink or shrivel up") describes an infant suffering from chronic and wasting child sickness who in fact wants to die.

33. Jane Ferguson, interview by author, Princeton Theological Seminary, Princeton, New Jersey, July 1997.

34. A. B. T. Byaruhanga-Akiiki and Obed N. O. Kealotswe, *African Theology of Healing* (Gaborone, Botswana: PrintWorld Ltd., 1995), 165–66.

35. "Health is a dynamic state of complete physical, mental, spiritual and social well being and not merely the absence of disease or infirmity." *World Health Organization,* 1998.

36. Larry Dossey, *Beyond Illness* (Boulder: New Science Library, 1984), vii.

37. Ibid.

38. Bernie S. Siegel, *Love, Medicine and Miracles: Lessons Learned About Self-Healing from a Surgeon's Experience with Exceptional Patients* (New York: Harper & Row, 1986).

39. Dossey, *Beyond Illness,* 109.

40. Robert G. Jahn, "Information, Consciousness, and Health," *Alternative Therapies* 2, no. 3 (May 1996): 38.

41. Mary McGarry, "Spirituality: A Growing Market Challenge," *Healthcare Marketing Report* 14, no. 12 (July 1996): 8.

42. A number of practices manipulate a person's energy field such as shiatsu, healing touch, and Reiki.

43. It should be noted, however, that some nurses such as members of the Christian Nurses' Association have taken a position opposing therapeutic touch because of its roots in Eastern religions.

44. Richard Jerome and Vickie Bane, "Touchy, Touchy," *People,* 27 April 1998, 93.

45. Ibid., 94.

46. Karen Philigan, "Therapeutic Touch: Using Your Hands for Help or Heal," in *Health and Faith: Medical, Psychological and Religious Dimensions,* 137.

47. Colt, "See Me, Feel Me, Touch Me, Heal Me," <http://www.pathfinder.com/Life/essay/altmed/altmed01.html>, 2 of 20 (24 November 1998).

48. Sandy Rovner, "Healthtalk: The Nurse's Touch," *Washington Post,* 2 December 1983, D5.

49. Jerome and Bane, "Touchy, Touchy," 94.

50. Larry Dossey, *Healing Words: The Power of Prayer and the Practice of Medicine* (San Francisco: HarperSanFrancisco, 1993), 47–48.

51. Ibid., 64.

52. Ibid.

53. Fitzpatrick, *Create Your Own Health Patterns,* 14.

54. William A. Nolen, *Healing: A Doctor in Search of a Miracle* (New York: Random House, 1974).

55. Leslie D. Weatherhead, C.B.E., "Present-Day Non-Medical Methods of Healing," in *Religion and Medicine*, 42–45.

56. Dossey, *Healing Words*, 197.

57. Fitzpatrick, *Create Your Own Health Patterns*, 60.

58. David Suzuki and Peter Knudtson, *Genethics: The Clash between the New Genetics and Human Values* (Cambridge: Harvard University Press, 1989), 297–99.

59. Dossey, *Healing Words*, 199.

60. Dale A. Matthews, David B. Larson, and Constance P. Barry, introduction to *The Faith Factor: An Annotated Bibliography of Clinical Research on Spiritual Subjects* (Rockville, Md.: National Institute for Healthcare Research, 1993), vol. 1, unnumbered pages.

61. Norberg and Webber, *Stretch Out Your Hand*, 20.

62. Dossey, *Healing Words*, 164–65.

63. For substantiation, see studies of David Moberg, Sol Levine, Andrew Greeley, J. J. Jackson, and W. R. Garrett cited in Elizabeth McSherry, "The Scientific Basis of Whole Person Medicine," *Journal of the American Scientific Affiliation* 35, no. 4 (December 1983): 218.

64. Ibid., 220. These were Protestant church–based primary health care clinics located in local church buildings.

65. Ibid., 222.

66. W. J. Strawbridge, R. D. Cohen, et al., "Frequent Attendance at Religious Services and Mortality over 28 Years," *American Journal of Public Health* 87, no. 6 (1997): 957–61; "Frequent Church Attenders Live Longer," research report, National Institute for Healthcare Research, Rockville, Md.

67. T. W. Graham, B. H. Kaplan, J. C. Cornoni-Huntley, S. A. James, C. Becker, C. G. Hames, and S. Heyden, "Frequency of Church Attendance and Blood Pressure Elevation," *Journal of Behavioral Medicine* 1978 (1): 37–43, in Matthews et al., *The Faith Factor*, vol. 1, 132.

68. McSherry, "The Scientific Basis," 222.

69. Andrea Neal, "Benefits of Religious Practice," *Indianapolis Star News*, 6 November 1997, Headlines: Andrea Neal's Commentary, <http://www.starnews.com/news/editorial/97/nov/1106SN neal.html> [30 October 1998].

70. H. G. Koenig, L. K. George, and B. L. Peterson, "Religiosity and Remission of Depression in Medically Ill Older Adults," *American Journal of Psychiatry* 155, no. 4 (April 1998): 536–42; "Spirituality Aids Recovery from Depression," research report, National Institute for Healthcare Research, Rockville, Md.

71. Matthews et al., "Methods," introduction to *The Faith Factor*, vol. 1, unnumbered pages.

72. Matthews et al., "Future Research Directions" and "General Conclusions," introduction to *The Faith Factor*, vol. 1, unnumbered pages.

73. Matthews et al., "Overall Trends," introduction to *The Faith Factor*, vol. 1, unnumbered pages.

74. Ibid.

75. Michael McGinnis and William Foege, "Actual Causes of Death in the United States," *Journal of the American Medical Association* 270 (10 November 1993): 2207.

76. Matthews et al., "Overall Trends," introduction to *The Faith Factor*, vol. 1, unnumbered pages.

77. J. S. Levin and H. Y. Vanderpool, "A Systematic Review of Findings Concerning Religious Commitment and Blood Pressure Status," *Social Science and Medicine* 29 (1989): 69–78, in David B. Larson, *The Faith Factor: An Annotated Bibliography of Systematic*

Reviews and Clinical Research on Spiritual Subjects, vol. 2 (Rockville, Md.: National Institute for Healthcare Research, 1993), 44.

78. J. J. Beutler et al., "Paranormal Healing and Hypertension," *British Medical Journal* 296 (1988): 1491–94, in Matthews et al., *The Faith Factor*, vol. 1, 29–31.

79. G. W. Comstock and K. B. Partridge, "Church Attendance and Health," *Journal of Chronic Diseases* 25 (1972): 665–72, in Matthews et al., *The Faith Factor*, vol. 1, 53.

80. D. R. Hannay, "Religion and Health," *Social Science and Medicine* 14A (1980): 683–85, in Dale A. Matthews and David B. Larson, *The Faith Factor: An Annotated Bibliography of Clinical Research on Spiritual Subjects*, vol. 3, *Enhancing Life Satisfaction* (Rockville, Md.: National Institute for Healthcare Research, 1995), 61.

81. C. K. Hadaway et al., "Religious Commitment and Drug Use among Urban Adolescents," *Journal for the Scientific Study of Religion* 23, no. 2 (1984): 109–28, in Matthews et al., "Religious Commitment and Drug Use in Adolescents," *The Faith Factor*, vol. 1, 138–39.

82. Dossey, *Healing Words*, 210.

83. Ibid., 40 ff.

84. Ibid., 128.

85. Ibid., 146–55.

86. Ibid., 185.

87. Ibid., 205.

88. Ibid., 207.

89. Paul Ramsey, *Fabricated Man: The Ethics of Genetic Control* (New Haven, Conn.: Yale University Press, 1970), 122–23.

3. DISCERNING AND DEFINING AUTHENTIC HEALTH AND HEALING MINISTRIES

1. George Santayana, American philosopher and critic (1863–1952), text unknown.

2. Steven Barrett, Arthur W. Hafner, and John E. Zwicky, eds., *The Reader's Guide to Alternative Health Methods* (Chicago: American Medical Association, 1993).

3. Shelly Fish of the Christian Nurses' Association is pursuing such studies.

4. Boston Associated Press, "Prayer and Prozac: Faith Healing Explored," *Trenton (New Jersey) Times*, 16 December 1996, A9.

5. Ibid.

6. McGarry, "Spirituality: A Growing Market Challenge," 7.

7. Ibid.

8. *Time*, 8 April 1996, 24 June 1996, 28 October 1996, 16 December 1996, 24 March 1997, spring special 1997, 12 May 1997; *Life*, September 1996, December 1996, December 1997.

9. McGarry, "Spirituality: A Growing Market Challenge," 9.

10. Ibid., 7.

11. Fitzpatrick, *Create Your Own Health Patterns*, 37.

12. Ibid., 35.

13. Ibid., 59.

14. Ibid., 58.

15. Erastus Evans, "The Significance of the New Testament Healing Miracles for the Modern Healer," in Crowlesmith, *Religion and Medicine*, 78–83.

16. McGilvray, *The Quest for Health*, 88.

17. Evans, "The Significance of the New Testament Healing Miracles," 82.

18. See Evans, *Redeeming Marketplace Medicine*, for section on Jesus Christ's healing ministry.

19. Norberg and Webber, *Stretch Out Your Hand*, 30.

20. Fox, *The Church's Ministry of Healing*, 16.

21. Weatherhead, "Present-Day Non-Medical Methods of Healing," 39; Leuven Institute lectures, 47; John B. Shopp, ed., *HarperCollins Encyclopedia of Catholicism, A–Z* (New York: HarperCollins, 1995). As we examine the whole faith healing phenomenon, one of the most famous sites of these healings is Lourdes, which for some epitomizes what is wrong with the faith-healing approach.

In 1858 a young girl of fourteen years of age had a number of visions of the virgin Mary at Lourdes, in the south of France. Mary directed her to dig in the earth, which she did, and a well sprang forth that has yielded water ever since. Since then millions of people have made pilgrimages to Lourdes for healing. Only a very small percentage claim physical healing, but many acknowledge peace of mind and acceptance, which they did not have before. Weatherhead, in examining the Lourdes phenomenon, more or less concludes that Lourdes has no therapeutic value.

This conclusion may be too harsh because many have testified to a variety of healings besides physical ones. In studies done the emotional impact of preparing and going to Lourdes seems to be a very important part of the process. People who were sick and marginalized become the center of attention, and much preparation takes place. Except for the original people who were healed, local people do not seem to be healed because all the emotional content is not present.

The Roman Catholic Church has established very rigorous criteria as to what events qualify for authentic healing; only 58 cases out of 5,000 reported miracles have been verified as authentic healing miracles at Lourdes.

22. Fox, *The Church's Ministry of Healing*, 92.

23. Weatherhead, "Present-Day Non-Medical Methods of Healing," 51.

24. Norberg and Webber, *Stretch Out Your Hand*, 22.

25. Maddocks, *Journey to Wholeness*, 157.

26. Gusmer, *The Ministry of Healing*, 24.

27. Pattison, *Alive and Kicking*, 50.

28. Ibid., 59.

29. Duncan, *Pastoral Care and Ethical Issues*, 128.

30. Ibid., 27.

31. V. Edmunds and C. G. Scorer, *Some Thoughts on Faith Healing*, 3d ed. (Rushden, Eng.: Christian Medical Fellowship, 1979).

32. Duncan, *Pastoral Care and Ethical Issues*, 14.

33. Health ministry definition used by author in her Lilly Health Ministry Research Project 1997–98.

34. *Beginning Health Ministry: A 'How to' Manual*, 3d ed. (Health Ministries Association, November 1995), 1-1.

35. Leuven Institute lectures, 30.

36. Norberg and Webber, *Stretch Out Your Hand*, 82 ff.; Michael Welker, *God the Spirit* (Minneapolis: Fortress Press, 1994).

37. R. A. Lambourne, "Wholeness, Community and Worship," in *Explorations in Health and Salvation: A Selection of Papers by Bob Lambourne*, ed. Michael Wilson (Birmingham, Eng.: University of Birmingham, 1985).

38. This quote was heard by the author at a lecture at Georgetown University in the 1980s.

39. See description of Stephen Ministries in chapter 10.

40. See chapter 8 for a description of the parish nurse program.

4. DEVOTIONAL, SACRAMENTAL, AND LITURGICAL PRACTICES

1. See Henri Nouwen's classic work on this subject, *The Wounded Healer* (Garden City, N.Y.: Image Books, 1979). Also see Evans, *Redeeming Marketplace Medicine*, for an extensive discussion of the problematic relationship of sin and sickness and the corrective to false correlations between them.

2. Gusmer, *The Ministry of Healing*, 119.

3. Maddocks, *Journey to Wholeness*, 158.

4. Maddocks, *The Christian Healing Ministry*, 19.

5. David Lee, "A Historical Sketch of Developments in the Church's Ministry to the Sick," in Gregg, *Ministry to the Sick*, 4.

6. Peter Fink, ed., *Alternative Futures for Worship*, vol. 7, *Anointing of the Sick* (Collegeville, Minn.: Liturgical Press, 1987).

7. Thomas A. Shannon and Charles N. Faso, O.F.M., *A Family Prayer Service to Assist in the Withdrawal of Life Support Systems*, n.d.; Sisters of Life, *Sisters of Life Healing Service for Abortion* (Bronx, N.Y.: Archdiocese of New York, n.d.).

8. *The Book of Common Prayer and Administration of the Sacraments and Other Rites and Ceremonies of the Church According to the Use of the Church of England* (New York: Henry Holt, 1994).

9. Duncan, *Pastoral Care and Ethical Issues*, 122.

10. Maddocks, *The Christian Healing Ministry*, 148.

11. Fox, *The Church's Ministry of Healing*, 70.

12. Frost, *Christian Healing*, 351.

13. Maddocks, *The Christian Healing Ministry*, 152.

14. Fitzpatrick, *Create Your Own Health Patterns*, 53 ff.

15. R. B. Byrd, "Positive Therapeutic Effects of Intercessory Prayer in a Coronary Care Unit Population," *Southern Medical Journal* 81 (1988): 826–29, in Matthews et al., *The Faith Factor*, vol. 1, 44–45.

16. Dossey, *Healing Words*, 69–70.

17. Ibid., 100.

18. Ibid., 98–100.

19. Ibid.

20. Ibid., 180, 185.

21. Ibid., 186, 165.

22. Daniel Benor quoted in Dossey, *Healing Words*, 189.

23. Dossey, *Healing Words*, 189–92.

24. Ibid., 195.

25. Weatherhead, "Present-Day Non-Medical Methods of Healing," 57–58.

26. William Strawson, "The Theology of Healing," in Crowlesmith, *Religion and Medicine*, 108.

27. See companion book, Evans, *Redeeming Marketplace Medicine*, for a discussion of this thorny problem.

28. David Watson, *Fear No Evil* (London: Hodder & Stoughton, 1984).

29. Ecclesiasticus 38:1–2 (NRSV): "Honor physicians for their services, for God created them; for their gift of healing comes from the Most High, and they are rewarded by the king."

30. Weatherhead, "Present-Day Non-Medical Methods of Healing," 57–58.

31. Frost, *Christian Healing*, 328.

32. Kelly, *Early Christian Doctrines*, 422 ff.

33. Duncan, *Pastoral Care and Ethical Issues*, 87.

34. Frost, *Christian Healing*, 308.

35. Lee, "A Historical Sketch," 10 ff.

36. Archbishop Michael Ramsey quoted by Maddocks in *The Christian Healing Ministry*, 114.

37. Fox, *The Church's Ministry of Healing*, 61.

38. Maddocks, *Journey to Wholeness*, 93.

39. Kelly, *Early Christian Doctrines*, 422 ff.

40. Maddocks, *The Christian Healing Ministry*, 123.

41. Frost, *Christian Healing*, 316.

42. Buchanan and Wheaton, *Liturgy for the Sick*, 5.

43. See Colin Buchanan, *Latest Liturgical Revision in the Church of England 1978–1984*, Grove Liturgical Study no. 39 (Bramcote, Eng.: Grove Books, 1984), 29–33, for a thorough discussion of this.

44. Maddocks, *The Christian Healing Ministry*, 121.

45. Carolyn Headley, *The Laying On of Hands in the Parish Healing Ministry* (Bramcote, Eng.: Grove Books, 1988), 3.

46. Gusmer, *The Ministry of Healing*, 118. Touching for the King's evil relates to a royal tradition of healing from scrofula (glandular disease).

47. Frost, *Christian Healing*, 332.

48. Church of England Central Board of Finance, *Ministry to the Sick* (Cambridge: Cambridge University Press; Suffolk: William Clowes [Publishers] Ltd.; Oxford: Oxford University Press; London: SPCK, 1983), 35.

49. Buchanan and Wheaton, *Liturgy for the Sick*, 20.

50. Church of England Central Board of Finance, *Ministry to the Sick*, 166–73. This is called the Public Service of Healing and includes anointing and laying on of hands.

51. Charles Harris, as cited in Gusmer, *The Ministry of Healing*, 124.

52. Buchanan and Wheaton, *Liturgy for the Sick*, 8.

53. See Lewis Smedes, ed., *Ministry and the Miraculous* (Pasadena, Calif.: Fuller Seminary, 1987), for an account of the Fuller controversy.

54. See story on pages 36–37.

55. Michael Perry, ed., *Deliverance: Psychic Disturbances and Occult Involvement* (London: SPCK, 1996), 100.

56. Frost, *Christian Healing*, 114.

57. C. S. Lewis, *The Screwtape Letters* (New York: Collins, 1972), quoted by Fox in *The Church's Ministry of Healing*, 22–23.

58. Welker, *God the Spirit*. See especially 195–219 for an insightful passage on demon possession.

59. Keir Howard, "New Testament Exorcism and Its Significance Today," *Expository Times* 96 (January 1985): 105–9.

60. *The Book of Common Prayer for Use in the Church in Wales*, vol. 2 (Church in Wales Publications, 1984), 770.

61. Ibid., 756.

62. *The Book of Occasional Services* (New York: Church Hymnal Corporation, 1994), 174.

63. Perry, *Deliverance*, 2.

64. Ibid.

65. Ibid., 12.

66. Maddocks, *The Christian Healing Ministry*, 127.

67. Bishop Morris Maddocks, interview by author, Chichester, West Suffolk, England, 26 October 1996.

68. Perry, *Deliverance*, 40 ff.

69. *The Book of Common Prayer for Use in the Church in Wales*, 770–71.

70. Perry, *Deliverance*, 44.

71. Ibid., 48.

72. Ibid., 71.

73. Norberg and Webber, *Stretch Out Your Hand*, 67.

74. Ibid., 79.

75. Ibid., 81.

5. EDUCATIONAL PROGRAMS

1. Abigail Rian Evans, "Saying No to Human Cloning," in *Human Cloning: Religious Responses,* ed. Ronald Cole-Turner (Louisville, Ky.: Westminster John Knox Press, 1997), 30.

2. Gena Corea, *The Mother Machine* (New York: Harper & Row, 1985).

3. Notes from author's independent seminar with Paul Ramsey at Princeton University, 1973. Determining one's position on definitions of death and dying is not the only issue in euthanasia. The very term "euthanasia" is a confusing one. In some ways, Ramsey may be right that "help in dying" (*Sterbehilfe*) as the German bishops refer to euthanasia (good death) is better. Even Arthur Dyck's term *bene mortasia* does not really solve the problem. However, his reference to our pledge to provide care for those who need it using the good Samaritan ideal of mercy is a good model.

4. Paul Ramsey, *Ethics at the Edges of Life* (New Haven, Conn.: Yale University Press, 1978).

5. Nancy Beth Cruzan, age twenty-nine, was in an automobile accident on January 11, 1983, leaving her in a persistent vegetative state. Her parents "sought authorization from a Missouri trial court to terminate her artificial nutrition and hydration." The U.S. Supreme Court in 1990 confirmed the decision of the Missouri Supreme Court, which had reversed a lower court's authorization of termination of treatment on the grounds that there was no "clear and convincing" evidence that Cruzan would have wanted to terminate her treatment. Subsequent to this, new evidence presented by her parents was deemed "clear and convincing" by a Missouri court, and Cruzan died in December 1990. (Bonnie Steinbeck and Alastair Norcross, eds., *Killing and Letting Die,* 2d ed. (New York: Fordham University Press, 1994), 79.)

6. Richard McCormick, Intensive Bioethics Course, Kennedy Institute of Ethics, Georgetown University, Washington, D.C., 1985.

7. This subject now requires separate texts for its discussion. See Robert F. Weir, *Physician Assisted Suicide* (Bloomington: Indiana University Press, 1997). In the spring of 1999, after repeated dismissals of charges, Kevorkian was convicted of second-degree murder.

8. Carol Gilligan, *In a Different Voice: Psychological Theory and Women's Development* (Cambridge: Harvard University Press, 1982).

6. SUPPORT AND ADVOCACY

1. Barbara Myerhoff, an anthropologist and critic of contemporary dehumanizing values in American mass culture, quoted by David L. Kertzer and Jennie Keith, ed., in "Rites and Signs of Ripening: The Intertwine of Ritual, Time, and Growing Older," *Age and Anthropological Theory* (Ithaca, N.Y.: Cornell University Press, 1984), 312.

2. Rhoda Halperin, "Age in Cultural Economics: An Evolutionary Approach," in Kertzer and Keith, *Age and Anthropological Theory*, 167.

3. Colin Brown, ed., *The New International Dictionary of New Testament Theology*, vol. 1 (Grand Rapids, Mich.: Zondervan, 1975), 193. Scripture offers many positive images of the elderly. The classic Greek words for "old" first signified older in relation to others and later to things of greater importance. In Plato's writing it referred to rank or dignity. In the Dorian world the preeminence that went with age led not only to a representative function abroad, but also to an advisory one within the political community.

Elders as rulers can be traced back to times of the Hebrew Scriptures—"elder of Israel"— and carried into the early church. The term *presbuterio* refers to greater length of life in Luke 1:18, Titus 2:2, and Philemon 9, which reminds us of Hebrew Scripture links between long life and virtue. For example, Presbyterians should have a built-in respect for the elderly since their name derives from the Greek *presbuterio*, which means "to be older, to be an ambassador, or to rule."

The use of these words in the Bible reflects the attitudes toward the various seasons of a person's life, so the fact that "Presbyterian" in its root meant "older" and then was expanded to connote "rule," "authority," "ambassador," reflects a point of view toward the young versus the old.

Another interesting word in the Christian Scriptures is *helikia*, meaning "age, life span, stature, or maturity." In Judaism there was great respect for older men (Lev. 19:32) because they had wisdom and understanding (Job 15:10). In Ephesians 4:13, maturity was the goal of the Christian. In fact, older people were so respected that Paul had to write Timothy not to despise his youth.

4. Henry Simmons, director of the Center on Aging Office, Presbyterian School of Christian Education, telephone interview by Jane Ferguson, research assistant, April 1997.

5. Karl Barth, *The Doctrine of Creation: Church Dogmatics*, trans. A. T. Mackay, T .H. L. Parker, Harold Knight, Henry Kennedy, and John Marks, vol. 3, pt. 4 (Edinburgh: T. & T. Clark, 1985), 607.

6. Ibid., 616.

7. *Chronic Care in America: A 21st Century Challenge*, 27.

8. Edwin Friedman, *Generation to Generation* (New York: Guilford Press, 1985), 150.

9. See Evans, *Redeeming Marketplace Medicine*, for a discussion of health care reform.

10. Deborah Harris-Abbott, ed., "The Lutheran Tradition: Religious Beliefs and Health-Care Decisions" (Chicago: Park Ridge Center for the Study of Health, Faith and Ethics, 1996), 2.

11. "Health Care: Lutherans Respond," n.p., n.d.

12. Ibid.

13. "American Baptist Resolution on Health Care for All," 8193: 11/91, facsimile provided 23 May 1997 by Office of Communication, American Baptist Churches USA, Valley Forge, Pennsylvania, 2.

14. Ibid.

15. "Universal Access to Health Care in the United States and Related Territories," in *Faithful Witness on Today's Issues: Health and Wholeness* (Washington, D.C.: General Board of Church and Society, The United Methodist Church, n.d.), 9.

16. Ibid., 9–15.

17. "Report of the Standing Commission on Health (1989–1991)," facsimile provided by Trinity Cathedral in the Episcopal Diocese of Pittsburgh, 179.

18. "Report of the Standing Commission on Health (1991–1994)," facsimile provided by Trinity Cathedral in the Episcopal Diocese of Pittsburgh, 289.

19. Ibid., 295–96.

20. Ibid., 293.

21. Subsequent quotations from this section are from "Executive Summary," in *Setting Relationships Right: A Proposal for Systemic Healthcare Reform* (St. Louis: Catholic Health Association of the United States, 1993), ix–x.

22. Ibid., x–xv. The section on Roman Catholics is based on material from the Catholic Health Association of the United States in 1993 in light of the situation at that time and may not necessarily hold true in 1999, according to Robert Stephens, Senior Associate, Communication Services.

7. THE CHURCH DELIVERS WHOLISTIC HEALTH CARE

1. See chapter 1.

2. *Chronic Care in America: A 21st Century Challenge*, 42, 64–65.

3. See Evans's companion book, *Redeeming Marketplace Medicine*, which discusses causes and places of death.

4. *The Search for a Christian Understanding of Health, Healing and Wholeness*, a Summary Report on the Study Programme of the Christian Medical Commission of the World Council of Churches 1976–1982 (Geneva: Christian Medical Commission of the World Council of Churches, 1982), 18.

5. Ibid., 27.

6. Ibid., 33.

7. Ibid., 21.

8. Press release (Washington, D.C.: Capitol Hill Wholistic Health Center, November 1982).

9. Capitol Hill Wholistic Health Center, Washington, D.C., brochure, n.d.

10. Norberg and Webber, *Stretch Out Your Hand*, 45.

11. Duncan, *Pastoral Care and Ethical Issues*, 67–72.

12. Donald Capps, *The Poet's Gift: Toward the Renewal of Pastoral Care* (Louisville, Ky.: Westminster John Knox Press, 1993), 1. See also Capps's other excellent books on pastoral care, such as *Pastoral Care and Hermeneutics* (Philadelphia: Fortress Press, 1984) and *Reframing: A New Method in Pastoral Care* (Minneapolis: Fortress Press, 1990), among others.

13. Julian of Norwich, *A Shewing of God's Love* (London: Sheed & Ward, 1958), 58. Julian of Norwich captures this perspective with real clarity: "For God is ever the same in love, but during the time when man is in sin he is so unmighty, so unwise and so unloving, that he can love neither God nor himself. The greatest defect that he has, is blindness, for he sees not all this. Then the holy love of God All-Mighty, that ever is one, gives him a sight of himself. At this he thinks that God is angry with him because of his sins, and then is stirred to contrition, and by confession and other good deeds to slake the wrath of God,

until he finds peace of soul and delicacy of conscience. It seems to him now that God has forgiven his sins, and this is true. The soul is made aware that God is turned to behold it, as if it had been in pain or in prison, saying thus: I am glad that thou art come to rest; for I have ever loved thee and love thee, and now thou lovest me. And thus with prayers and with other good works that are customary, according to the teaching of Holy Church, is the soul owned to God."

14. Duncan, *Pastoral Care and Ethical Issues*, 64.

15. See, for example, Howard Clinebell's illuminating writings, such as *Understanding and Counseling Persons with Alcohol, Drug, and Behavioral Addictions* (Nashville: Abingdon Press, 1998), *Ecotherapy: Healing Ourselves, Healing the Earth* (Minneapolis: Fortress Press, 1996), *Counseling for Spiritually Empowered Wholeness* (New York: Haworth Pastoral Press, 1995), and *Well Being* (San Francisco: HarperSanFrancisco, 1992), and the work of Richard Gilbert at the World Pastoral Institute, 1504 N. Campbell, Valparaiso, Ind. 46385.

16. Deborah van Deusen Hunsinger, *Theology and Pastoral Counseling: A New Interdisciplinary Approach* (Grand Rapids, Mich.: Eerdmans, 1995), 5.

17. Ibid., 215.

18. Maddocks, *The Christian Healing Ministry*, 167.

19. Gusmer, *The Ministry of Healing*, 92 ff.

20. "Clinical Theology," *Health and Healing*, no. 41 (September 1996): 1, Churches' Council for Health and Healing, London.

21. Ibid., 2.

22. Duncan, *Pastoral Care and Ethical Issues*, 107.

23. Herbert Benson with William Proctor, *Your Maximum Mind* (New York: Times Books, 1987).

24. The Reverend A. Philip Parham, *The Church and Alcohol: A Resource Manual*, S-4. No update of this statistic is available.

25. See Cecil Williams, *No Hiding Place* (San Francisco: HarperSanFrancisco, 1992), for a church that is a place of refuge and change in the Tenderloin District of San Francisco. See chapter 10 for more information on this ministry.

26. Stephen P. Apthorp, "Drug Abuse and the Church: Are the Blind Leading the Blind?" *Christian Century* 105 (9 November 1988): 1010.

27. *Addiction: The Churches' Responsibility*, Christian Medical Commission of the World Council of Churches (Celigny, Bossey, Switzerland: Ecumenical Institute, March 1988), 6.

28. Hilary Abramson, "Alcohol Giants Market Misery to 'Third World,'" *Marin Institute for the Prevention of Alcohol and Other Drug Problems*, newsletter, no. 12 (winter 1997): 2, <http://www.marininstitute.org/NLSP97.html> [13 November 1998].

29. Ibid.

30. Ibid.

31. J. Madeleine Nash, "Addicted: Why Do People Get Hooked?" *Time*, 5 May 1997, 71.

32. Clemens Bartollas, *Juvenile Delinquency*, 4th ed. (Needham Heights, Mass.: Allyn and Bacon, 1997), 335.

33. "Economic Costs of Alcohol and Drug Abuse," NIH News Release, National Institutes of Health, 13 May 1998, 1–2 <http://www.nih.gov/news/pr/may98/nida-13.htm> [3 June 1999].

34. Robert M. Weinrieb, M.D.. and Charles P. O'Brien, M.D., Ph.D., abstract, "Naltrexone in the Treatment of Alcoholism," *Annual Review of Medicine 1997* 48: 477–87 <http://biomedical.AnnualReviews.org> [8 December 1998].

35. *NCADD Fact Sheet: Alcoholism and Alcohol-Related Problems* (New York: National Council on Alcoholism and Drug Dependence, 1995), 1, 3.

36. "Youth, Alcohol, and Other Drugs: An Overview," National Institute on Drug Abuse (NIDA), 1996 National Household Survey on Drug Abuse <http://www.ncadd.org/youthalc.html> [17 November 1998].

37. "Youth, Alcohol, and Other Drugs: An Overview," National Institute on Drug Abuse (NIDA), Drug Use among Racial/Ethnic Minorities, 1995, 31 <http://www.ncadd.org/youthalc.html>, 1 [17 November 1998].

38. *NCADD Fact Sheet: Youth and Alcohol* (New York: National Council on Alcoholism and Drug Dependence, 1996).

39. Ibid.

40. Bartollas, *Juvenile Delinquency*, 330.

41. Ibid., 330–31.

42. Ibid., 332–33.

43. "Substance Abuse—a National Challenge," U.S. Department of Health and Human Services Fact Sheet, 20 December 1997 <http:/www.health.org/mtf/hhsfact.htm>, 2.

44. "Facts about Teenagers and Drug Abuse," National Institute on Drug Abuse, September 1997 [NIDA Capsule—Monitoring the Future Study <http://www.health.org/pubs/caps/NCTeenagers.htm>, 1.

45. "Substance Abuse—a National Challenge," 2.

46. Gerald May, *Addiction and Grace* (San Francisco: Harper & Row, 1988), 24.

47. Ibid.

48. Ann Wilson Schaef, *When Society Becomes an Addict* (San Francisco: Harper & Row, 1987), 18, 29.

49. Ibid., 26.

50. May, *Addiction and Grace*, 83.

51. *Alcohol Use and Abuse: The Social and Health Effects*, Reports and Recommendations by the Presbyterian Church (USA) (Louisville, Ky.: Office of Health Ministries, Social Justice & Peacemaking Ministry Unit, Presbyterian Church [USA], 1986), 35.

52. See Linda Mercadante, who attempts to bring these models together in *Victims and Sinners: Spiritual Roots of Addiction and Recovery* (Louisville, Ky.: Westminster John Knox Press, 1996).

53. Hans Selye, *The Stress of Life* (New York: McGraw Hill, 1976), 1.

54. Leo Goldberger and Shelomo Breznitz, eds., *Handbook of Stress: Theoretical and Clinical Aspects* (New York: Free Press; London: Collier Macmillan, 1982); Joseph D. Matarazzo et al., eds., *Behavioral Health: A Handbook of Health Enhancement and Disease Prevention* (New York: Wiley, 1984), 44, which lists twenty stress factors.

55. Chris Schriner/exercises by Sue Ingels Mauck, *Feeling Great: Practical Psychology and the Christian Faith* (Peoria: Wesley Kolbe Publishers, 1986).

56. "High on the Job," *Washington Post*, October 1989, health section, 13.

57. Carole Rayburn, Lee Richmond, and Lynn Rogers, "Stress Among Religious Leaders," *Thought* 58, no. 230 (September 1983): 342.

58. Robert Weigl, *Hayfield Secondary School Stress Survey: Final Report* (Fairfax, Va., June 1984, photocopy).

59. Adapted from the book *Type A Behavior and Your Heart* (New York: Knopf, 1974) by Meyer Friedman, M.D., and Ray Roserman, M.D.

60. Benson, *Your Maximum Mind*, 92–95.

61. LynNell Hancock with Debra Rosenberg, Karen Springen, Patricia King, Patrick Rogers, Martha Brant, Claudia Kalb, and T. Trent Gegax, "Breaking Point," *Newsweek*, 6 March 1995, 56–62.

62. Ibid., 60.

63. Ibid., 58.

64. "High on the Job," 13.

65. Nouwen, *The Wounded Healer*.

66. Lambourne, "Wholeness, Community and Worship," 20.

67. When I was serving on the Commission on Values for the Washington, D.C., Board of Education in the late 1980s, this truth was brought home to me. After almost a year of meeting, this group of educational experts decided that what were needed to break the cycle of violence, teenage pregnancy, drug use, and school dropouts were adults who mentor and work with the kids on a one-to-one basis, not a curriculum.

68. Presbyterian Church (USA) Network on Alcohol and Other Drug Abuse, *The Congregation: A Community of Care and Healing* (Louisville, Ky.: PCUSA, 1990).

69. Abigail Rian Evans, "Drugs: Everybody's Problem," *Presbyterian Survey*, April 1990, 27–28.

70. *Alcohol Use and Abuse: The Social and Health Effects*, 35.

71. Walter Shapiro, "Essay," *Time*, 18 September 1989, 104.

72. See chapter 10 for more information on this program.

8. PARISH NURSING—A NEW SPECIALTY

1. This more definitive task is being accomplished by the International Parish Nurse Resource Center in Chicago, and potentially by the members and elected officials of the Health Ministries Association whose information is based on firsthand experience as practitioners in the field.

2. Norma Small and Abigail Rian Evans, "Parish Nurses as Integrators of Health" (paper presented at the annual Parish Nurse Conference, Chicago, Illinois, September 1989), 19.

3. Ibid., 20.

4. Ibid.

5. Ibid.

6. Joan Zetterlund, "Kaiserwerth Revisited: Putting the Care Back into Health Care," *Journal of Christian Nursing* 14, no. 2 (spring 1997): 12.

7. Ann Solari Twadell, interview by author, December 1997, International Parish Nurse Resource Center, Chicago, Illinois. There are five thousand on their mailing list, but because of the loose use of the term "parish nurse," it is difficult to determine exact numbers.

8. "History of Parish Nursing," bookmark, International Parish Nurse Resource Center, Chicago, Illinois.

9. Practice and Education Committee of the Health Ministries Association, Inc., *Scope and Standards of Parish Nursing Practice* (Washington, D.C.: American Nurses Publishing, 1998).

10. Anne Marie Djupe, RNC, M.A., "Documentation: Tracing Our History-Underlining Our Future," *Perspective in Parish Nursing Practice* 3, no. 4 (Park Ridge, Ill.: Parish Nurse Resource Center, winter 1993): 4. Of course, it is true that as the parish nurse movement has matured, they too are required to provide documentation for their work.

11. Granger E. Westberg, "The Church as Health Place," *Dialog: A Journal of Theology* 27 (winter 1988): 191.

12. The Parish Nurse Resource Center, Park Ridge, Illinois, and the national Health Ministries Association, with offices throughout the United States, work with the ANA to interpret the standards.

13. *Scope and Standards of Parish Nursing Practice*, 15–22.

14. Granger E. Westberg and Jill Westberg McNamara, *The Parish Nurse: How to Start a Parish Nurse Program in Your Church* (Park Ridge, Ill.: Parish Nurse Resource Center, 1987), 11.

15. Ibid., 61.

16. Some of these functions are mentioned in *Beginning a Health Ministry: A "How to" Manual*, ed. Maureen Ahrens and Joni Goodnight, produced by the Health Ministries Association, 3d ed., November 1995, funded by a grant from Lutheran Brotherhood Foundation, Minneapolis, Minnesota, containing photocopied materials from many sources around the country, and in the International Parish Nurse Resource Center material on the functions of the parish nurse.

17. Anne Marie Djupe, RNC, M.A., Harriet Olson, RN, M.S.N., Judith A. Ryan, RN, Ph.D., FAAN, with Jane C. Lantz, *An Institutionally Based Model of Parish Nursing Services* (Park Ridge, Ill.: International Parish Nurse Resource Center, n.d.).

18. Joni Goodnight, facsimile to author, 21 January 1999.

9. STARTING A HEALTH MINISTRY

1. Carl Geores, retired director of Ministries in the North Country (MINC), Maine, "The Start of a Housing Ministry," draft (20 November 1996), 2; Carl Geores, *Resource Book for Building Church and Community Ministries* (Princeton, N.J.: Princeton Theological Seminary, 1997).

2. Drawn from ideas in Geores, "The Start of a Housing Ministry," 6–7.

3. Duncan, *Pastoral Care and Ethical Issues*, 120.

4. Much of the information that follows is based on the very practical *Beginning a Health Ministry: A "How to" Manual*.

5. Upon request the author can provide a list of health ministry resource organizations.

6. Williams, *No Hiding Place*, 23.

7. See Westberg, *Theological Roots of Wholistic Health Care*, for one of the early discussions on wholistic health.

8. Kent C. Miller, June Begany, Harold Clark, and John Sharick, *The Staywell Program Handbook: A Health Enhancement Program for Church Professionals* (Louisville, Ky.: Presbyterian Church [USA], n.d.), 1–2; see chapter 9, Evans, *Redeeming Marketplace Medicine*, for further development of this theme.

9. See Evans, *Redeeming Marketplace Medicine*, chapter 9, for a discussion of this section.

10. *Beginning a Health Ministry: A "How to" Manual*, 3-1, 2.

11. Ibid., 4-17.

12. See Suzanne Farnham, Joseph P. Gill, R. Taylor McLean, and Susan M. Ward, *Listening Hearts: Discerning Call in Community* (Harrisburg, Pa.: Morehouse Publishing, 1991).

13. *Beginning a Health Ministry: A "How to" Manual*, 4-1, 2.

14. Maddocks, *The Christian Healing Ministry*, 148–50.

15. Norberg and Webber, *Stretch Out Your Hand*, 89, 91.

16. Maddocks, *The Christian Healing Ministry*, 148–50.

17. "How Your Church Can Have a Ministry of Counseling and Healing" (Kingston, Jamaica: Jamaica Baptist Union Counseling & Healing Ministry Committee, n.d.), photocopy, 3.

18. The Guild of St. Raphael, *The Ministry of Healing: An Anglican Contribution* (Penrith, Cumbria: Reed's Ltd., n.d.), inside cover.

19. D.S. Allister, *Sickness and Healing in the Church* (Oxford: Latimer House, 1981). The entire book discusses scriptural texts on healing.

20. Geores, "Building Your Own Model for Cooperative Ministry: A Bible Study Process," Bible Study Guide, in *Resource Book for Building Church and Community Ministries.*

21. *Beginning Health Ministry: A "How to" Manual,* 4-1, 2.

22. *The Staywell Program Handbook,* 6–7.

23. Maddocks, *The Christian Healing Ministry,* 148–50.

24. *Beginning a Health Ministry: A "How to" Manual,* 4-1, 2.

25. *1993 Annual Report,* Church Health Center, Memphis, Tennessee, 20.

26. The Acorn Christian Healing Trust in England offers such training called "Christian Listeners."

27. *Beginning a Health Ministry: A "How to" Manual,* 4-3.

28. Williams, *No Hiding Place,* 23.

29. Ibid., 8–10.

30. Based on Geores, *Resource Book for Building Church and Community Ministries.*

31. Donald Smith, *Congregations Alive: Practical Suggestions for Bringing Your Church to Life through Partnership in Ministry* (Philadelphia: Westminster Press, 1981).

32. Thomas Droege, the Carter Center Health Ministries in Theological Education Conference at Columbia Theological Seminary, handout, Decatur, Georgia, April 1997.

33. Ibid.

34. *Beginning a Health Ministry: A "How to" Manual,* 3-1.

35. Ibid., 3-1, 2.

10. PRACTICAL PROGRAMS FOR HEALTHY PEOPLE

1. Maurine Trautz Nelson and Abigail Rian Evans, *Directory of Health Ministries Models,* National Capital Presbytery Health Ministries (Washington, D.C.: E. F. Printing, 1988).

2. See 62–69.

3. *Contact* (Christian Medical Commission, World Council of Churches), no. 113, February 1990.

Credits

From John Fitzpatrick, *Create Your Own Health Patterns* (Dublin: Mercier Press, 1980). Reprinted by permission. • The section in chapter 6 on Roman Catholics is based on material from the Catholic Health Association of the United States in 1993 in light of the situation at that time and may not necessarily hold true in 1999, according to Robert Stephens, senior associate, Communication Services. Reprinted by permission. • From Dale A. Matthews, David B. Larson, and Constance P. Barry, introduction to *The Faith Factor: An Annotated Bibliography of Clinical Research on Spiritual Subjects* (Rockville, Md.: National Institute for Healthcare Research, 1993), vol. 1, unnumbered pages. Used by permission. • From telephone interview with Robert Ellis, associate for program development and resourcing, International Health Ministries Office of Worldwide Ministries, Division of Presbyterian Church USA, Louisville, Kentucky. Used by permission. • From telephone interview with Henry Simmons, director of the Center on Aging Office, Presbyterian School of Christian Education. Used by permission. • From Norma Small and Abigail Rian Evans, "Parish Nurses as Integrators of Health" (paper presented at the annual Parish Nurse Conference, Chicago, Illinois, September 1989). Used by permission. • From Morris Maddocks, *The Christian Healing Ministry* (London: SPCK, 1981). Used by permission. • From Tilda Norberg and Robert Webber, *Stretch Out Your Hand: Exploring Healing Prayer,* copyright © 1990, United Church Press, Cleveland, Ohio. Reprinted by permission. • From John Crowlesmith, "Non-Medical Healing from the Age of the Fathers to the Evangelical Revival," in *Religion and Medicine,* ed. John Crowlesmith (London: Epworth Press, 1962). Used by permission, • From Evelyn Frost, *Christian Healing: A Consideration of the Place of Spiritual Healing in the Church of To-Day in the Light of the Doctrine and Practice of the Ante-Nicene Church* (London: A. R. Mowbray & Co., 1940). Last known copyright 1940 by

Index

The healing church : practical

320030101442754

Printed in the United States
27317LVS00005BA/1-18

9 780829 813401